Gabrielle Morrissey, PhD has been a sexologist-sexuality educator, sex consultant and sex researcher-since 1990, and has worked in sex therapy, education and research in many countries, especially Australia, Britain, and the United States. In addition to her lectures and workshops which she delivers around the world, Dr. Gabrielle runs university courses in sexology and heads her own sexology consultancy program, Bananas and Melons (www.bananasandmelons.com.au). Currently based at Bond University as Assistant Professor, she teaches a stream of four human sexuality subjects across two academic programs. Dr. Gabrielle also serves as Adjunct Associate Professor in the Division of Health and Applied Sciences at Southern Cross University.

Also by Gabrielle Morrissey

Urge : Hot Secrets for Great Sex
Sex in the Time of Generation X

A Year of
Spicy Sex

52 RECIPES

TO HEAT UP YOUR SEX LIFE

Gabrielle Morrissey, PhD

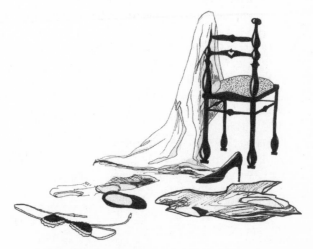

Marlowe & Company
New York

A YEAR OF SPICY SEX:
52 Recipes to Heat Up Your Sex Life

Copyright © 2006 Bananas and Melons Pty Ltd

Published by
Marlowe & Company
An Imprint of Avalon Publishing Group, Incorporated
245 W. 17th Street, 11th Floor
New York, NY 10011-5300

AVALON
publishing group incorporated

Originally published as Spicy Sex: 52 Sumptuous and Saucy Recipes for Red-Hot
Loving Every Week of the Year in Australia by HarperCollins Publishers in 2006.
This edition published by arrangement.

Library of Congress Cataloging-in-Publication Data

Morrissey, Gabrielle.
  A year of spicy sex : 52 recipes to heat up your sex life / Gabrielle
Morrissey.
      p. cm.
  ISBN-13: 978-1-56924-262-9
  ISBN-10: 1-56924-262-3
  1. Sex instruction. 2. Sex customs. I. Title.
  HQ31.M727 2006
  613.9'6--dc22

                                        2006014344

9 8 7 6 5 4 3 2 1

Printed in the United States of America

Dedicated to
lovers and lovees
the world over

A Year of Spicy Sex

Acknowledgments

This book is a product of much passion and practice, and not just mine. I owe a great debt of gratitude to the many unnamed couples, and partners, who tried out recipes and supplied ingredients, tips and techniques over the time it took to develop and create this book.

In addition, I'd like to thank a few specific people who contributed help to the book, and to me, as I was writing it. Thank you so much for your support: Nick, Peter and Di Morrissey, Nicole David, Lily Brooker, Lollie Barr, Jodie Bradnam, Bec Agg, Sandy Macken, Chauby, Igor Persan, Duncan Hardman, Lydia Barnes, Amanda Lambros, Dwone Jones, Lyndell Crawford, Sophie Hamley and Alison Urquhart. Cheers!

Basics

To Start . . .

This recipe book is for your bedroom and beyond. The recipes in each section are designed to give you ideas for varied, exciting, sensuous and delicious sex. You can adapt them to suit your own tastes, or you can follow them exactly for a bit of saucy fun. Each recipe provides details of setting, preparation, ingredients, recommended techniques, positions, play, talk . . . all the way through to boiling-hot orgasm delivery.

When it comes to food, we crave variety. Yes, most people have dishes that are their favorites, but if we ate the same thing day in and day out—so that it was our sole sustenance—we'd eventually get bored and desire it less. With food, we sample many different dishes. People regularly try new recipes, alternate cuisines and learn new twists on old standards. In many ways, the same principles can be applied to our sex life: variety keeps it interesting and stimulating. Many people get a little worried about adding a bit of spice to their sex life. "Will it have to involve leather chaps, whips and wax?" they nervously think to themselves. "I thought clamps were for woodworking!" they squeak, their voices laced with a touch of anxiety, to the saleswoman in the sex shop.

In reality it's not only possible, but more successful, to revolutionize your sex life through a series of small changes, rather than leaping headlong into the land of radical sex. This recipe book for spicy sex is about achieving added sexual excitement through realistic measures—nowhere will you find a suggestion such as "greet your partner at the front door wearing nothing but saran wrap!"

While you might not find every suggestion or technique practical or particularly appealing for you, consider the ideas in each recipe as inspiration for your own sexual resourcefulness. Sustainable change, in any context, is best achieved through a series of small steps over time. Spicing up your sex life doesn't mean suddenly trying something well beyond your comfort zone. Simply trying one new thing can bring about a world of difference to your perception of intimacy, and inject your libido with a higher energy. Increasing the passion between you as a couple can be as straightforward as changing one aspect of your sexy time together just once a month, or breaking one routine. If at the present time you don't pay too much attention to setting a mood, for example, taking a bit of effort to light some candles or to create a color or aromatic theme can significantly transform a sexual experience. It doesn't take much time or preparation, and yet the rewards can be manifold.

Sexuality is a fundamental aspect of our identity and expression, so even the slightest investment in your sex life can have multiple payoffs, for you and your partner.

Burning Passion
Many couples reach a point when they ask, "Why don't we have the same passion we had at the beginning of our relationship? What happened?" They can blame each other, their lifestyles, their domestic situation, their work commitments, fatigue, lack of time, and more—however, few couples are educated about the nature of passion: that it

isn't designed to last. That's right—passion is not designed to last in the same bubbling, silly, nervous, hyperventilating way it feels like when people first fall into that cascade of lust and love.

When we first meet, and experience the flush of lust and, perhaps, of falling in love, our bodies are actually pumping with "love chemicals," the most powerful of which is phenylethylamine (PEA), which is responsible for those undeniable feelings of fluttering excitement when we see our partner—our knees go weak (literally), our palms sweat, we get butterflies in our stomach, we "ping" at them whenever they appear in our sphere, and concentration on anything else is a total loss. The very stuff expressed timelessly by poets and troubadours. It's a very inefficient state for the body to be in, and yet it's determinedly designed to get us to meet, mate and (potentially) procreate. As such, the longest it ever really lasts in anyone is about 18 months, and very often less.

Initial passion is biochemical and ignited during the partner-discovery process. Once that's been experienced, that same kind of passion can't be regained. Passion, in its essence, boils down to us "clicking." The "sticking together" part isn't about passion so much as commitment, determination, decision, bonding, emotion, action, planning and behavior. You can regain a certain amount of exciting passion, but it won't be the same kind of passion you had at the very start of your relationship. Partly this is because of a lack of PEA, and partly it's because the intimacy you've developed means you have to redefine excitement, and "discovering each other" means reaching deeper into your fantasies and intimacies, and rediscovering why you fell for each other through expression of feelings, appreciation and desire in the same, and new, ways.

This rediscovery or reinvention process in a relationship can be very illuminating, and is an exhilarating time for any couple. Couples who sustain passion over time do so through growing together and maintaining a sexual, emotional and spiritual connection through that growth. Couples who feel connected intimately in the bedroom, who are sexually satisfied, tend to fight less, nag less, communicate more effectively and feel more united as a couple.

As a rule, people generally underestimate the role of sexual intimacy in a relationship. We take sexual function and pleasure for granted until it breaks down, and then it causes great distress. Often it's only at this point that couples—or singles—address sexual concerns. By maintaining a varied and spicy sex life across the life span of a relationship, people can prevent many sexual problems.

Many couples split over sexual issues: infidelity, low sexual desire, sexual incompatibility, or a lack of pleasure, fulfilment and appreciation. It's natural for couples, and singles, to go through sexual highs and lows, but prioritizing sexual intimacy in a relationship can prevent many sexual problems, including boredom, perfunctory sex or infrequent sex. A varied sex life is essential to maintaining a high libido, and to remaining connected as a passionate couple.

Your most important sexual organ is the one between your ears, not the one between your legs. Your erotic brain is the key to good sex, because it processes all five senses, tells you you're turned on and is the instrument of desire. When you stimulate your mind, and your partner's mind, by giving your sex together a bit of extra attention, the rest of your erogenous self, from tip to toe, responds.

One of the secrets to a passionate, long and happy intimate relationship is to keep sex on the front and center of your brain, and the recipes in this book can be used to achieve that goal by helping you to vary your sex life, rediscover your lover, try new techniques, romance your partner, and keep the sexual part of your relationship on the front burner of the stove, rather than letting it slide to the back burner, then off the stove, until it's out of the house entirely and frozen in the back fridge out on the rear veranda! It takes much more energy to heat up a sex life that has perhaps quietly and slowly chilled than one that keeps its own heat-seeking momentum by virtue of regular pinches of spice.

The Five P's

Is it hard to spice up your sex life? Honestly, no. It takes a few simple principles to stimulate or sustain the passion in a relationship, a little bit of time and some creative ideas, which are suggested throughout this book for you. The primary principles boil down to the Five P's:

Priorities—make sure your intimate time, for just the two of you alone, is a priority, not just an activity at the bottom of your list to resort to when you can squeeze in the time. Intimacy is a necessity in a successful, satisfying relationship.

Playfulness—sex for procreation is the minority expression of our sexuality. Over a lifetime couples will have far more sex for recreation. Sex is your adult playtime, so have fun with it! Sex doesn't always have to be a soap opera seduction, so laugh, giggle, play games, tease and please.

Pleasure—sex and intimacy is about pleasure, not necessarily about orgasm. Focus on the giving and receiving of pleasure, rather than the goal of orgasm, for a total experience of physical and emotional pleasure.

Pampering—we're more in the mood for sex when we feel good and have the energy for sex. Sex takes time, concentration and some effort, so in order to be primed for pleasure, take time out for yourself. De-stress, exercise, do things to make yourself feel sexy and sensual: beauty care, massages, cologne, fashion, sport and hobbies. Investing in yourself and your sexiness will pay off in your sex life.

Partner connection—research has revealed that good sex is about feeling connected to your partner. Sex is a shared activity, so make sure you feel connected with your partner outside the bedroom as well as between the sheets. The more you feel like a couple in life, the more you'll feel connected and satisfied in passionate coupling.

And then, practice, practice, practice!

Sexy Health Benefits

This recipe book is designed to help you create passionate, red-hot stimulation in your sex life. In this day of fatigued jugglers, dual-income and hard-working couples, stress is one of the biggest libido killers, and the distress call for "more sex, please" or "more excitement and passion, please" can often be met with a sigh or a groan (and not the sexy kind, either). This is such a common occurrence that the phrase DINS has been coined to label the phenomenon: DINS = Double Income No Sex.

"Just use a little bit of imagination!" cry sexologists, but it's entirely understandable if you're tapped out of ideas or don't have the spare energy to be creative and imaginative when "maintenance sex" is the maximum you can muster. People are busy—reading this, you might find that this resonates with you, so, go ahead and nod—and the struggle to satisfy the wish for a happy quantity of sex in your life can often win out over the ability to satiate your desire for the highest quality of exciting sex on a week-to-week basis.

Or maybe you don't resonate with the DINS scenario at all. Perhaps you have a brilliant sex life, and you want to ensure it stays that way. Good for you! Top marks for a healthy choice. The recipes in each section can serve in the "good-to-great" model so that, even if your sex life isn't flagging in the least, there is still a bevy of ideas and techniques to keep your sexual chemistry sparking with variety and thrill.

Sex is important, not only because we love it, but also because it is Good For You. Unlike traditional cookbooks in which most of the truly delicious recipes have not-so-good-for-you ingredients, all of the recipes in this book are 100 percent healthy for you ... and calorie-burning too!

Sex is one of our most basic drives, just behind the need for food and shelter. It has some very primal benefits: physical, emotional and spiritual. Physically, sex is good for your heart—literally! Lovemaking is good aerobic exercise, and the sexual response keeps your circulatory system toned and healthy. Sexually active people suffer fewer heart attacks. Sex can also be good for your waistline, as foreplay and intercourse can burn anywhere between 150 to 550 calories ... depending on how active you are and long you go for! (It's certainly a more entertaining way to keep trim than the treadmill.)

The sexual response also provides a measure of pain relief—endorphins released during orgasm make us feel "high" and can relieve pain from various conditions, including arthritis, backache and headaches. No more headache excuse to get out of sex—sex can actually cure a headache! There is also some research to show that sex even has a positive wellness effect on people in ill health, particularly those with cancer. Initial studies suggest that oxytocin and the hormone DHEA, both released through orgasm, may prevent breast cancer tissue cells from developing tumours. And in men, ejaculation keeps the prostate gland healthy and helps prevent prostate cancer by halting the build-up of toxins and carcinogens. Sorry, guys, but this is not based on daily ejaculations—you only need a few a month to benefit.

In terms of a positive effect on our emotional and mental states, sex provides a plethora of neurochemicals released at orgasm which help make us feel good, and the sensation of touch can alleviate depression (mild, not clinical—if you suffer from depression do not stop taking medication and use sex as your sole health tonic). Hormones released during the sexual arousal response act as disinhibitors, ease fears and anxieties, and increase a sense of calm and well-being.

Perhaps one of the best benefits we get from sex is its healthy effect on the toll stress can take on us. The times we are stressed are when we most often neglect or turn away from sex, but this is precisely when we could be using sex as a health aid to reduce stress. Regular sexual expression, including intercourse, boosts immune cells, reduces physical and emotional stress, and helps us fight off illness. Use the recipes in this book as your stress-busting sex diet!

Even with the compelling case for sex being good for you, some couples still resist the idea that a healthy sex life should take structure, work, investment and time. Satisfied or not, many people think that "sex should just be natural, shouldn't it? No thought, no planning, it's just instinct, isn't it?" But this is one of the biggest myths about sex, full stop.

Of course sex is natural, and if you want a lifetime of "basic bonks" like many other animals in nature, you may be happy thinking that there's nothing more to learn. But humans are more evolved and complex than other animals, and our emotional link to sexuality is very important. So while sex is absolutely natural, an active pursuit of learning more about our holistic sexuality—including fulfilment, function, expression and enhancement—across our changing relationships, identities and lives, is just as natural.

So learning about sex, and ever expanding your interest in keeping it varied and passionate, is natural and good for you, and many couples long for the opportunity to do all of that ... if only they could find the time. This book is specifically designed to help cut down on already existing stress levels and increasing time debt by providing detailed recipes that leave nothing to chance—and, thus, nothing to stress over! Across 52 recipes, a wide repertoire of sexual options is presented, leaving virtually nothing for the imagination alone to conjure.

Substitutions

While the Kama Sutra is most often considered the "bible of sexual pleasure," perhaps the second most recognized and appreciated sex book is the ultra-famous *The Joy of Sex* by Alex Comfort. It was he who famously compared sex to cooking, sectioning his book into topics such as "sauces," "ingredients" and "main courses." Since his concept was first published, some sexologists have continued to compare the need to feed the appetites; however, it is still taboo, even in a new millennium, to experiment as widely with sex as we do with food.

A Year of Spicy Sex encourages you to explore your appetite for new sexual experiences without any judgment about or boundaries around personal taste. Unlike most food recipe books which require strict adherence to ingredients and process, this recipe book is yours to own and adapt, to suit the individual, private and unique sensuous satisfaction of you and yours. Indulge yourselves and add your own substitutions to the recipes, tweak them to suit you and use them as a springboard into a whole new approach to investing in your sex life. You can use these recipes to enhance your sex life one night a week for a whole year—from anniversary to anniversary perhaps—or you can treat yourselves to a delicious gluttony of pleasure in a short space of time. These recipes might give you ideas for even more recipes of your own creation.

It's important to note that while most of the recipes in this book specifically refer to hetero-sex, many of the techniques can be easily substituted for use with same-sex partners. Find the portions that turn you on, and adapt and enjoy together, for whomever you're indulging with! Also, none of the recipes strictly adhere to the principles and practice of "safer sex." If you are in a non-monogamous relationship, are unsure of your partner's sexual history or need to use precautionary measures, please include your individual latex additions accordingly. It's especially important that you substitute latex-friendly lube whenever oil is called for in a recipe, as most oils can cause damage to latex. The recipes are

meant to serve as spice to your sex life, but are not intended
to sabotage safety.

Spice Up Your Sex Life

There are a total of 52 recipes in this book, so each week for
an entire year there is something new to spice up your sex
life. There are six sections, and while some of the recipes in
each section require a little more planning and preparation,
others are ideas to boost spontaneity and fun. After all, spicy
sex is our adult fucking fun time!

The six sections reflect varying appetites and a wide cuisine. From Nibbles through to Hot, Sizzling, Quick & Easy,
Sweet and Gourmet, there are recipes for long, lazy, rainy
Sundays when you can make love all afternoon, and for fervent sneaky sex, when ravenous desire captures you and you
cannot wait, you have to have your lovee then and there, for
just a few fiery minutes.

Nibbles

Before getting too excited about "spicing up your sex life,"
it's important to ask and answer the question "What is sex?"
It may seem obvious, but it's not. As a society we generally
define sex as PV, or penile-vaginal, intercourse. When we talk
to our friends and lovers about sex, many (not all) assume
that this is what is meant. But is sex really confined to this
narrow definition? Of course not. Sex is about far more than
intercourse, and to view sex as being only penetrative intercourse is a limiting and narrow definition of human sexual
expression. Sex encompasses the vast, wide spectrum of
human sexual experience, which includes intercourse but is
not limited to it. This is important when considering the

variety of people's sex lives, and sexual desires and fantasies. People can be ultimately, fantastically, sexually satisfied without having experienced intercourse.

Currently, we have too much emphasis on sex as a goal-oriented sport. We're so focused on the skill of "scoring" to the goal of orgasm, preferably for both parties, simultaneously, with her then multiplying her head off, that we've lost appreciation for the entire journey of pleasure.

The recipes in this book, especially in the Nibbles section, place the focus back on the pleasure of the whole sexual, sensual experience, instead of tracking single-mindedly towards orgasm and intercourse. Every now and then it's important to connect sexually without creating a pattern of intercourse, so that when you do touch each other sensually the fluttering zing is there, and the notion of "perfunctory sex" is zapped from your sexual communication. So, enjoy your Nibbles with each other—go back to "making out" from time to time and watch your sexual desire for each other really start cooking!

Hot

From Go to Oh-oh-whoa, these recipes walk on the wild side, but always with realism and a bit of naughty fun. Some offer practical tips, tested and suggested by a variety of couples, such as how to have sand-free, or sand-minimal, beach sex, and others show how to make the most of middle-of-the-night sex, outdoor "or bush" sex, and making love to music.

Sizzling

Cross the wild side and enter a world of sexual adventures.

Become absorbed in your fantasies, your partner's fantasies, develop a sexual alter ego and create erotic experiences you've been curious about but never (yet) tried, or learn how tiptoeing into the world of bondage and domination can release the Master or Mistress in you.

Quick & Easy

Ardent. Intense. Impatient. Unforgettable. The "quickie" may have earned a bad reputation as inferior sex because of its naturally short duration and because women rarely experience orgasm in those few minutes—however, the quickie is actually a staple of many couples' sex lives. Granted, the quickie is not designed for maximum female pleasure, but try out these recipes to help women achieve orgasm, and increased arousal, even during a quickie, and experience quickies so greedy and hot that the excitement created in the "have to have you" moment is adrenaline-pumping thrill enough.

Sweet

Here's the truth: both men and women report wanting to have more sex . . . and more romance. Romantic sex is lovely. Yes, it takes time and energy to create a warm ambience, but the appreciation and attention feel so good that the smiles and bonding it creates last days and days, long after the sex itself is over. These recipes are for those indulgent times when you want to really lavish love.

Gourmet

Enrich your sex life by taking the extra time to spoil your partner with loving delights on those special occasions throughout the year. For birthdays, Valentine's Day, anniversaries and holidays, treat your partner to thoughtful touch. Take these days together as a "celebration of us."

Those are the basics. From here the planning, prioritizing and preparation are up to you."Spicing up your sex life" used to be a vague statement. Now it has specific recipes. Healthy, good-for-you, satisfying recipes.

Indulge and enjoy.

Satiate yourselves until you are replete with pleasure.

Nibbles

*A lot can be said
in a breath.
I want
language to
produce beauty,
touch to punctuate,
taste to tell the tale.*

Lollipop Lickstick

A red-hot blow job to blow his mind.

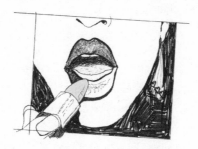

Pleasure Pantry Ingredients
Red lingerie, including suspenders
Red lipstick
Chair
Skirt

Preparation
Get into the seduction of the color red. While, statistically, more women prefer wearing black lingerie, the color men most prefer to see a woman wearing is red. Engage your inner red vixen and let it out for this red-hot, blow-his-mind blow job.

Red is a powerful color, especially on lips, because, according to anthropologists, as soon as lips are heightened in red—especially a red that happens to match lingerie men can see—the lips become a "genital echo," serving as a not-so-subtle association with your *other* pair of sexy, enticing lips. They become entrancing, and his awareness of them is often quickly followed by a rush of blood to his genitals, accompanied by an immediate heat of desire.

The only preparation needed for this Nibble is to be wearing your red lingerie and to coat your lips in heavy red lipstick—really overdo it because, this time, you want it to come off ... all over him. Pick a time and place that suits you, and then initiate ...

Bring to Boil

Sit him down on a chair and straddle him. Slowly reach down and raise each side of your skirt to reveal your hose and suspenders. Don't kiss him but instead take his hands and, with your own, guide his fingers to feel what you're wearing under your skirt. Then take one of his fingers and suck it, leaving a light lipstick ring around the base of it.

With a sexy smile, scoot off his lap and onto your knees. Pull his legs apart, reach in between them and unzip him. Before you put your mouth on him, hike your skirt up to around your waist so he can see not only your face in his lap but also get a view of your butt and thighs encased in sexy red lingerie. This "revealing of the hidden" while you orally pleasure him will stimulate his visual senses and his naughty fantasies. You can show him even more of your bum if you kneel over him from the side. Either way—full frontal or view from the side—move your hair so he can see your face and mouth as you're on him. Men love to watch—especially when you're having your way with him and leaving your mark.

Open your lips wide and take him in your mouth, to the base of his shaft. Close your mouth around him and seal him with a lipstick stamp. Leave a dark ring of lipstick encircling him, then smear it upwards. As you move up and down, licking and sucking him, the lipstick can tinge his whole shaft, especially if you added gloss after applying your lipstick. The lip color might also smudge on your mouth and face, but don't worry about how you look—messed-up lipstick is like sexy bed-hair: it proves you're concentrating more on what you're doing than what you look like. Your face smeared with red lipstick can feel messy, wild—even slutty. Embrace it. "Slutty" is a momentary adjective, not an identity.

Give him head using a variety of mouth and tongue movements—monotony is definitely not the name of this game. Tease the head of his penis with flicks of your tongue, then vary this action with long, hard sucks and short, fast bobs. Kiss his sac, too. Go all out, have a ball, paint the testicles red!

If you get uncomfortable on your knees, try to shift your weight sexily so you don't break the magic you're creating for him by distracting him with something as real as sore knees. Instead, take an opportunity to give your knees and mouth a mini-break by hoisting yourself up onto his lap as if you're going to straddle him and take him inside you—but don't. Instead, stretch up and graze your nipples across his lips, both areas are sensitive, so it's pleasure for him and for you. Stopping to redirect his attention can frustrate him, but if it's quick—and if you do it with an intensity that shows you are really horny and really desirous of him, rubbing your body up and down his body—then returning your mouth to his dick transfers the insistence of the sexual momentum you're creating and will fire him up further.

Pull your lingerie down a little and touch yourself. Let him see you do this, but don't let him touch. Finger your wetness, then spread it on his chest to prove to him how much you're getting turned on by pleasing him. Slide back down his body, take him in your mouth again and make some noise as you suck him. Enhance the visual and tactile stimulation with some pleasing sound because, if he knows you're loving it, he's going to love it even more. The crescendo of stimulation will have him popping in ecstatic spasmic convulsions in no time.

Extra Zing

Do it in front of a mirror so he can see you from all angles, giving him hot 3-D delight. If you're worried at all about how your body looks, remember this: he's not watching your body, he's watching your mouth and the lines of the lingerie, and your hands, and your face. If you're still a little shy, though, switch off the lights and place a candle in the corner of the room. The candle can hide the parts of your body you perceive to be unsightly, yet throw enough light that the effect of the lipstick still sears.

If you want to add even more spice, try giving him the Lollipop Lickstick somewhere in semi-public (blow jobs in public view of anyone are illegal, though). But be prepared to emerge looking very sexed-up in your lipstick-smeared face! Channel an unabashed sassiness about it, and get your lover to show his appreciation by kissing off the rest of the lipstick smudge from your lips. Hold his hand and rub the lipstick you left on his finger earlier to remind him where else it still lingers.

Peaches and Cream

Eat her sweetness.

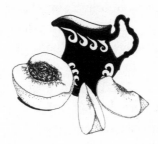

Pleasure Pantry Ingredients
Sliced peaches
Cream
Vibrator (optional)

Preparation
Many couples view oral sex as a foreplay technique rather than the main meal, which it deserves to be. Spend this time on your lovee indulging in every luscious part of her body, rather than diving down immediately for a low-down encounter as a top primer to penetrative climax. Make sure she knows that this session is all about having her as your delicacy. Get her in the mood to receive by lying her down and murmuring to her that you're going to please her, and that she need not return the favor—in the next ten minutes, or the next ten weeks. This experience isn't about exacting a give-receive ratio between you but is, rather, a gift of simple pleasure.

Bring to Boil

Once she's lying down and in the mood for receiving some loving, start by telling her how beautiful she is, and how erotic you find her body. Tell her that you love touching her, that giving her pleasure brings you pleasure. Many women have body insecurities and can feel uncomfortable receiving total attention directly on their body. Given the pressures women feel about looking ever-youthful and perfect, any acute attention to her body can put her on the edge of anxiety, especially because she's often trying to look her best for you in just these kinds of moments.

The critical self-talk women engage in can actually serve as a powerful off-switch for the arousal process and her sexual response, preventing her from enjoying your touch. You can redirect these potential worries of hers by heading her off at the pass with a flurry of compliments about her body parts. Some women aren't comfortable accepting compliments, though, so give her loving praise in a monologue as you kiss her body, rather than face-to-face compliments that might require a response. Allow her to just hear, and let her body respond naturally.

Start your celebration of her body by giving her a short, light massage, touching all over her body by skimming your fingers along her skin. Light touches are good for places where the skin is thin and rich with nerves, or in a spot that isn't used to being touched by another, such as inside the upper and lower arms, eyelids, ears, the backs of knees and hands, the scalp, back of the neck, jawline, and even armpits.

Once her skin is tingling from your touch, let your hands wander down towards her mound and below, to her outer and inner lips. Give her some hand stimulation on her vulva before leaning over to kiss her down below.

After a bit of lip brushing and nibbling, use your lips to create suction on different parts of her lips and clit. The contrast of your hot, soft lips and firm vacuum pressure will be highly pleasurable to her. While sucking you can also flick your tongue, but make sure you don't suck too hard. And go easy with your teeth: grazing, yes; biting and chewing, no. Spend a concentrated amount of time on her clitoral love button. There are 8000 nerve endings there, and they are twitching to be touched.

One of the greatest misunderstandings men make when it comes to orally pleasing a woman is thinking that it's the equivalent of a male blow job. Men often like oral—and nothing but oral—pleasure. Many women, however, like the contrast of the heat of the mouth and the soft, velvety touch of the tongue with the firm pressure of the finger and hand. Just as you might like to be brought to orgasm with fast, steady rhythmic motions, so does she, and sometimes these are best brought about by your hand, with your mouth as the added accentuation.

Create excitement through unpredictable touch—as soon as you create a pattern of pleasure with your tongue, highlight it with a finger touching her lips, or her clitoral shaft, that flexible cord-like love-line just above her clitoral button.

Just when she's writhing with glee, add some extra stimulation to her wetness by eating her with extra ingredients. Take a slice of peach and slither it between her lips. Use its natural wetness to further lubricate her, and excite her with its slippery sensation. The combination of the peach slice and your tongue will have her quivering with pleasure at the intense erotic combination of two similar yet slightly different wet and thick sensations on her increasingly wet nether regions.

If your tongue starts to get tired (which is common) give it a rest by pouring a little bit of cream onto her vulva. Help satisfy your voracious appetite for her by spreading the cream all over her with your fingers, across her mound, inner thighs, and the peachy crease of her bottom. The slippery wetness of the cream and juice will have her grinding for more stimulation. Go back down on her using a variety of long, slow licks alternating with hot, flat flicks of your tongue; and, also using your finger on her clit, bring her at last to orgasm, with your face following her swaying, shifting hips as she reaches climax. Spread the cream and peach juice around her inner thighs and pelvis, even up to above her pubic area, and when she's sighing and satiated, repeat your fervent moves to bring her to a second and third course.

Extra Zing

For added variety, use a vibrator to increase stimulation and decrease the amount of time it takes to get her to come. Don't rely just on the vibe, though—use it as an added accessory. In between your licks and sucks, place it against her clit and inner lips then remove it and return to tongue stimulation. The sensation of hard and intense pressure alternating with your soft and warm kisses will boost her mindful erotic sensation, and also cause her physical response to hiccup between racing and slowing, which will swell her sexual response so that, when she does come, the sweetness is ecstatically throbbing and explosive.

Kitten Heels

A purr-fectly erotic massage for him.

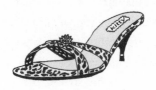

Pleasure Pantry Ingredients
Lingerie (crotchless optional)
Kitten-heeled shoes
Massage oil
Music (optional)
Candles
Hot, damp towels (optional)

Preparation
Put on lingerie and kitten heels. You can wear any sexy shoes, really, but not something so high that you can't move around in them. Aim to wear lingerie that has a peekaboo middle underneath so he can see teasing glimpses as you touch him during the massage. You can also rub him with your pussy, not just your hands, to make him absolutely quiver with excitement.

Most of the time during an erotic massage, his eyes will be closed. But that doesn't mean that for the moments when he is watching, you can't provide him with a visual feast that shows him your pussy and all the other body parts you're loving him up with.

Choose a room for the massage. It may be your bedroom, or you may wish to set up a makeshift massage table by laying plump pillows along a table for him to lie on. If he's lying in a position that enables you to lean over and massage him without climbing on top of him, you can then reach across and touch him without putting your weight on him, and it allows him to look over and eye you at navel and lingerie height when the desire strikes him.

Set the mood by putting on some music, if you wish, and lighting some candles. Candlelight allows you to see what you're doing but also keeps the room dark enough so he can relax and float away.

Tell him that the next hour is devoted entirely to him and making him feel good. All he needs to do is let go and receive your touch; his body needs only to simply react to that touch. He may orgasm; he may not. He may get hard, or he may not. He may get aroused and then lose it to total relaxation. This is a sensual, rather than sexual, massage so there is no pressure to perform.

Bring to Boil

Start with a light, scratching scalp massage. Some men hardly ever get them and can have intense reactions of pleasure. It's a good way to get a man to drop into instant relaxation, especially if his muscles are a bit tense from work, stress, deadlines, or just the sight of you circling or leaning over him wearing nothing but peekaboo panties and heels.

Encourage the impression of this being a sensual massage by avoiding his groin area for at least the first fifteen minutes—

it might take him this long to de-sexualize the experience and fall into relaxation mode.

Using the massage oil, give him some long, body-length strokes from his neck, along his back, across his bum and down his legs. Create a rhythm with these body strokes, on both sides.

Slowly increase the eroticism by paying some attention to his feet. If he hasn't had a shower and his feet are a bit ripe, get some hot damp towels (pre-heated) and wrap his feet in them while you continue a few more body strokes. Then start a foot massage. Gently and lightly touch the feet, trying not to tickle them, but engage them enough to stimulate the nerves there. The feet-related nerve receptors in the brain are near those for the genitals and some experts believe there is a neural pathway between these areas, so stimulation of the feet may inspire arousal in the genitals. Or if your lovee is easily ticklish, try reflexology of the feet, focusing on deep, slow touches on the toes, ball of the foot and inner arch, which are linked to the brain, heart and genitals respectively.

Massage up the legs and into the inner thighs. Give him a firm massage over both of his butt cheeks—this is a major muscle area, and one men frequently work out during sex, so it's a nice change of pace for him to receive sensual touch from you while this area remains relaxed. If you know he likes a deep-tissue massage, press more firmly. Some men get quite ticklish, though, so pay attention to his body reactions in order to alter your touch if need be.

From here, really start working into his lower back. Give him some acupressure on his sacrum, which is just above his tailbone—pressing the sacrum brings blood to the area and increases and enhances erection. Nine inches above his tailbone lies an area with a complex network of nerves that are connected to his genitals. Your goal is not to create an erection, necessarily, but he'll feel the benefits of this blood flow when he turns over and you work on his front.

Once you've spent a sufficient amount of time massaging his back, neck and shoulders—key areas where men hold a great deal of stress—give him a kiss on his neck and whisper to him to roll over.

Once he's lying on his back, work your hands into his shoulders again, and down his arms, spending time alleviating any tension in his biceps and triceps, which are the muscles in the upper arm. Give him some indulgent, soothing touches in those areas where men rarely get touched: his fingers, the palms of his hands, his toes and his face. Unless he's a metrosexual (booking into salons for regular pampering), he won't be familiar with how deeply wonderful it can feel to be massaged across his forehead, temples, cheeks and chin. Work your way down his chest, into his hips and down onto his thighs. Work into his inner thighs and then upwards towards his penis. This is a time when you can really explore his body and see how he responds to various types of touch, and it's best if his penis is soft or semi-erect so that you can try several playful ways to touch this very sensitive area. Roll his penis between both your hands, working up and down. This isn't a "hand job" (unless you or he want it to be at this point), so don't think of your touch as having to lead him to orgasm. Feel free to wander away from the penis down to the perineum (the spot between the genitals and the anus)—even to the anus if you wish, and back up to the scrotum. Circle your finger and thumb around the top of his sac and cup it with the other hand. Creating heat here with your hands will automatically lead to his balls pulling away from his body, and you can tug down on his scrotum—some men will find this slows down their sexual response, while others may find it completely arousing. Then massage his shaft liberally with oil and, if you want, add stimulation by blowing on him.

At this point, follow the mood—if you sense (or he tells or indicates to you) that he wants to come, you can continue to knead him until he ejaculates. Because it's a sensual rather than sexual massage, and you're the one dictating the touch, this might be a time when you can experiment with speed and rhythm to learn first-hand which kind he responds to best. At this point, though, some men will be so relaxed that coming won't be necessary at all. A kiss, a thank you and a snooze are all that will be in order.

Extra Zing

To add a bit of sexual touch to the sensual massage, straddle your lover as you massage his front. Create some different sensations for him by lightly brushing your hair across his face, down his neck and along his chest. Wearing your sexy undies that flaunt your pussy, rock your hips forwards and backwards along his navel area, and then along his legs. He'll get pleasure from the knowledge that the touch he's feeling isn't from your fingers but from your lower lips. Run your pussy along his shaft, then directly switch that touch back to your hands. This erotic massage may be fun, fondling touch, but it isn't a foreplay technique. When you're both spent, and he's fully relaxed from this downtime, click off in your kitten heels and tell him it's 100 percent okay on this occasion if he simply rolls over and goes to sleep.

A Slice of Heaven

A sensual massage to put her on cloud nine.

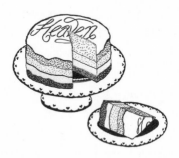

Pleasure Pantry Ingredients
Towels
Music
Candles
Incense or oil burner
Scarf
Wide-tooth comb
Soft hairbrush
Brush with soft bristles
Massage oil
Hot, damp towels (optional)
Heating pad (optional)
Hot water bottle (optional)

Preparation

For a total body and mind escape, set up the room to enhance all her senses. Whether you're going to massage her on the bed, or on pillows laid across the floor, right before inviting her in to lie down, tumble a few towels in the dryer so they're hot and spread them on the massage area so that when she does lie down she's enveloped in warmth. You may even add a few hot-water bottles or heated pads under the towels. Encourage her to adjust them to places that feel good for her.

Put on some soft music and light a few candles—just enough so that you can see, but leaving the room dark enough so that she can relax. Light some incense or an oil burner with a relaxing aromatherapy scent such as lavender or ylang ylang, or a scent you know she loves.

Tell her that the next hour is about pampering her; that you are there to help her relax and feel wonderful. Tell her to switch off her mind. Tell her that she doesn't need to think about anything for the next hour—everything is taken care of. She doesn't need to think about work, children, family members, the house or any other obligations. This hour is entirely for and about her. Tell her that, even though she's naked and you adore and desire her, this time is for her to receive your touch, there isn't any pressure to respond sexually—she is simply to go with the flow. She is to surrender and relax and not feel that she needs to please you back. Whether by the end of the hour she is aroused or asleep, the goal has been met—because there is no goal save enjoying the experience and the time-out.

Bring to Boil

Once you've invited her to lie down, start by giving her some long, loving strokes down the length of her back. Then lightly draw your fingers from her head to her toes, including a touch on her arms and hands. Starting this way creates a chemistry of touch along her whole body, so that from the beginning every exposed part of her has received some touch and she can relax, because she's not anticipating touch on any particular part of her body.

Before relaxing her with a traditional massage using oil, stimulate her skin with a scarf. Lightly skim the scarf along her body from her neck, down her arms, her back, across her bottom, down her legs, and then drape it down her feet. This light touch will bring her awareness to her skin's outer layer, and surprise her with a tingling sensation from tip to toe.

Next, take a wide-tooth comb, preferably with rubber or soft tips so they don't scratch or hurt, and further stimulate her skin by stroking the comb down her body in the same pattern you used with the scarf (if her feet are ticklish, avoid this and stop at her ankles). Take a few extra minutes to comb her hair, ending with a scalp massage, which will really help to drop her into a relaxation zone. Then, using a soft hairbrush, brush her hair. Women often love to have their hair brushed because it feels very nurturing, and as women generally are the primary nurturers, receiving nurturing touch can be wonderfully indulgent. To expand on this sensation, take a soft brush that has velvety-soft bristles and lightly brush her all over. The combination of sensations created will have her aching for deeper touch. Her skin will feel alive, awake and in love with the idea of touch.

Before you begin massaging her with oil, whisper to her and ask her to imagine that her muscles, and the deeper parts of her body, haven't been touched or pleasured for a long time. Ask her to visualize that this is the first time in a long time that her body has been indulged with any kind of touch. Having her think about and visualize parts of her body as if they haven't been touched in a long time can help her appreciate the power of your touch, and imagine how lovely it would feel if your contact, right now, was the first time her body had ever been touched. Every fiber of her will be amped up, anticipating this wondrous feeling.

From here you can indulge in firmer touch, with oil, all over her body. Spend at least twenty minutes massaging her neck, shoulders, arms, hands, back, bottom, legs and feet. Once you've touched and soothed every exposed part of her, lean down and whisper to her that it's time to turn over.

When she's lying on her back, start with the scarf, as you did before, to make her tingle all over. Be aware that the front of a woman's body can be more ticklish than the back, so use your judgment about where, and how lightly, you sweep the scarf over her. When she's alight with skin sensation, sedate the sensation by giving her scalp a deep finger massage. Then treat her to a facial rub. Most women who have facials often do so for skin-beneficial reasons, so to be treated to a purely tactile facial massage will feel wonderful. Give her small circular rubs along her forehead and the rim of her eyebrows, down to her temples, across her cheekbones, down through her cheeks, across her jaw line and to her chin. Lightly stroke down her throat and over to her ears, stimulating her outer ears and pulling on her lobes.

Add oil to your palms and massage down her upper chest to her breasts. Lightly circle her nipples and flick them a little—they're likely to become instantly hard because they are often sensitive to touch, but don't (as much as you may want to) dwell on the breast massage part of this experience. Communicate to her, nonverbally, that you really are there to pleasure all of her, and not to excite yourself, by playing with her breasts.

Lightly massage down to her navel, without tickling her, and then start a circular massage on her mound of Venus.

Using one finger, stroke down the length of each of her outer lips. Her outer and inner lips are rich with nerve endings, so even the lightest touch will elicit a throbbing, erotic response. Vary your touch down towards the entrance of her vagina, and outwards into her pubic muscles. Working on pressure points here will alleviate tension and help to relax her whole groin area—a touch she might not be used to, but might also really like.

If, at this point, she gives you an indication (or you ask her) that she'd like to come, stimulate her clitoral shaft, hood and glans, fast and slow, up, down and around, until she reaches orgasm. Resist your urge to penetrate her, even with one finger. Stay with external stimulation. Don't make this wonderful, erotic, sensual massage culminate in a penetrative sexual experience; this nibbling, massaging, pampering experience is about her needs and loving her body, not about foreplay extending into penetrative intercourse of any sort. Everything she needs to come is on her outside. Even if you know she loves internal stimulation, this particular experience is about variety, and making her come without internal touch. And, with oil on your hands, it's best not to enter her vagina, as many oils can interfere with the natural pH of the vagina. Once she comes (if she does or wants to), give her a kiss, cover her up to warm her, and tell her to drift off to blissfulness.

Extra Zing

For added spice and stimulation for you both, engage in some genital-on-genital massage. While massage is usually considered to be hand-on-body touch, use your penis to stimulate her body once she is lying on her back. Straddle her and massage her breasts with your hands, while your penis tickles her navel area. Then take your penis in your hand and rub it up and down on her vulva. If you're so excited that you release some pre-cum, take a finger and spread your wetness up and down her clitoris to provide lubrication to stimulate the head of her clit. Since you're not going to enter her—because this is nonpenetrative play—use your erection to stimulate her inner and outer lips. The psychological thrill for her, knowing that this is all about external play, will have her curiously wet until she comes. Be her clitoral climax cupid, shooting her up to cloud nine!

Pearl Delight

A pearler of a job for him.

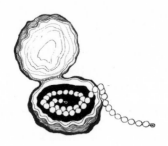

Pleasure Pantry Ingredients
White lace bra and panties
A strand of real pearls
Massage oil

Preparation
Fulfil the "good girl gone naughty" theme by wearing white lacy knickers and bra. Accessorize your lingerie simply with one strand of pearls around your neck. While it was mentioned earlier that most men prefer to see red on a woman, a huge proportion of them also love to sexualize the classic color of purity and see their lover wearing white while doing something deliciously, overtly sexual to them.

There is no preparation needed for the Pearl Delight, except to have a strand of real pearls at hand. It's important that your pearls are real, because fake pearls can often have lines or joins on them which can scratch or hurt your man, instead of teasingly pleasing him.

Bring to Boil

Invite your lover into the bedroom and, once he is lying down on the bed, prop him up with pillows so he's at an angle where he can see you play with him. The power of the pearls is not just tactile, but also visual. Sitting next to him, lean over and give him some kisses, but don't let him take any initiative to control this sexual scene: this is your time to be in control.

The juxtaposition of you being nearly nude, in white (domination is usually associated with black), yet being domineering, will spark his curiosity, and his arousal.

Many women don't initiate sex or many kinds of sexual play, especially hand jobs, because the pleasing is all in your hands and some women feel like they're "competing" with his masturbatory skill. So if you're one of the many for whom this is true, really extend this session to demonstrate that, yes, you are the one in control and, yes, you are the giver this time. Remember: the penis is your friend. Think of it as your playmate, not some alien creature that judges you with its every fluctuation. This is your chance to play with him, and if you feel a bit unsure, bear this in mind: as much as he may like to play with himself, he loves it when you do too, and you can be sure he's never done it with a strand of pearls in his hands!

Start the visual reward by unclasping your pearls from around your neck. If you need his help to do this, lean down and ask for it with a kiss and a smile. Before taking him with the pearls, twirl the pearls down your own body to focus his attention. Wrap them into a ball and massage them over your clit through your panties. Run them back up your stomach, across your navel and up to your breasts. Reveal a nipple and, with the other hand, twist the pearls around a finger and rub your nipple with them. Then wrap the pearls around your hand, across your palm, and reach down to his penis.

Since you've only just started, he might still be soft—and that's okay. Some women feel a sense of performance pressure if his dick doesn't automatically respond to the sight of them, but don't worry ... it will be hard in a minute, have confidence in that.

Run the pearls down and then up the length of his shaft, towards the head, to start him twitching with arousal. Then take the pearls from your hand and loop them around the base of his penis. Give him one or two strokes just with your hands, and then take the pearls in your hand and rub up and down him, using the pearls as the stimulant. Get him to notice the difference between this and a "regular" hand job—the pearls will create a soft, round, smooth, ribbing effect.

Lean over and put a smidgin of massage oil in your hands to allow for some lubrication, to create heated slipperiness as you continue to work on him. It's important—for the health of your pearls—that you use a light oil, rather than a moisturiser that contains perfume or alcohol, which can damage the delicate pearls' luster.

With the pearls wrapped around your hands, begin a basket-weaving motion up and down him. Clasp your hands and rhythmically knead up and down his shaft, right up to and including the head, twisting your wrists in a circular motion to really maximize the effect of the rotating pearls on his skin. Alternate this motion with straight up-and-down pumping, with both or one hand.

Take the pearls from your hands and encircle his penis with them, rubbing up and down. When you feel he's getting close to orgasm, keep going with the pearls or, if your man likes a hard and fast finish, wrap one loop around the base of his dick (like a cock ring), hold it tight, and with the other hand feverishly pump until he comes. He might take slightly longer than usual, with the ring of pearls squeezing the base of his penis, but that prolonged pleasure exactly before he orgasms will increase the pleasure-pulsing sensations when he does let go. When he comes, lift the pearls off of him, drape them back around your neck (taking a moment to wipe the oil off of them to protect them) and wear them for at least the next 24 hours to remind him, and you, of the experience.

Extra Zing

Enhance your pearl job by playing with his twin set. As you continue your vigorous motions up and down his shaft, remove the pearls and circle the top of his sac with them. Use them as a looped "catch" to tug down on his scrotum—gently. This will slow down his sexual response, and also increase his arousal. Lightly scratch his scrotal skin with your nails and then return your attention to his dick, while also cupping and fondling his balls with the pearls. Just when he's about to come, lean over and let him ejaculate on your neck, leaving you with an entirely erotic "pearl necklace" which he'll appreciate even more than your real pearl necklace . . .

The Gift of Love

Grant her the gift of time.

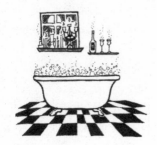

Pleasure Pantry Ingredients
Clock
Box and wrapping paper
Her favorite cocktail
Plate of her favorite appetisers
Bubble bath gel
Music
Candles
Book (one that she's reading, or has been wanting to)
Shampoo, conditioner, soap, loofah, soft sponge
One piece of chocolate
Card (optional)
Pamper/beauty vouchers (optional)

Preparation
Research suggests that when asked "Which would you prefer: a good night's sleep or sex?" almost half of all women opt for the snooze rather than the screw. This isn't to say that women don't want sex, but many of them crave sleep even more.

The old joke goes that "washing dishes is foreplay!" and this is because women feel they need a break from time to time. If anything is going to get them in the mood for lurve, it's a demonstration that you're there to help share the burden of daily duties. It's exhausting to be the partner, mother, career mogul, cook, domestic goddess and vampy sex goddess every day of every week of every month on end. A chance to relax and simply be a woman with some precious time alone can work wonders for her sense of sexiness, and also her libido. Whether your lady regularly fights fatigue-induced low libido or not, an evening of sex-free loving attention can top up her passion stores in just one night.

To really treasure your lovee, and have her feeling full of love for you and how wonderful you are, give her a loving evening that allows her to rest, relax and rejuvenate. The rewards you receive will include a grateful appreciation that can translate to a "yes"—rather than a yawn—next time you initiate sex with her. Don't give her this gift of time alone as an IOU. Rather, tell her that this time is simply for her. Acknowledge that indulgent time alone is important to her, and anything that's important to her is important to you.

To prepare for this evening, buy a little clock, place it in a box and wrap it as a gift. Then choose a night when you can make sure all other distractions are taken care of: there are no pressing deadlines the next day, the children are away for the night (or you take care of them), and take the phone off the hook. Create a "Do Not Disturb" atmosphere.

Bring to Boil

Start the evening early, so you can give her the entire night to relax. Get her attention by telling her that you have a gift for her. Present her with the clock in a wrapped box. When she opens it she might be a little puzzled, so with a smile explain to her that you're giving her "time." Sit her down, pour her a drink, offer her a plate of her favorite appetizers and tell her to relax, because everything is taken care of and for the entire evening her every whim will be attended to.

Run a bath for her. As the tub is filling, ask her how her day was. Focus the conversation on her, and listen to what she has to say. Try not to let the talk switch to being about you or your day, because you want to emphasize that tonight is all about her.

Pour plenty of your newly purchased bubble bath gel in the water and don't be stingy—use a liberal portion so that the bath is absolutely brimming with bubbles. This will seem luxurious to her, and make her feel spoiled and special. Put on some soft music, and adorn the bathroom with loads of candles; set her current (or "been meaning to get to this") book next to the tub. If it's winter, put a heater in the bathroom to create an enveloping warmth that she can unwind in.

Invite her in and slowly undress her. Make sure you take off her watch, because in giving her the gift of time, you release her from any knowledge of how long she's taking for herself. Ask her to get in the bath and sit yourself on the edge of the tub. Scoop bubbly water all over her body and head; take the suds in your hands and rub her back. Because this night is about total relaxation, don't even go near her front. Don't rev her up, or give her the impression that this night is one with sexual expectations, by touching any of her erogenous zones.

Take the shampoo and slowly, gently wash her hair. When a woman experiences nurturing touch from her lover that isn't sexual or even particularly sensual, that is purely caring and adoring, her heart will smile for you.

After this worship of her, tell her that you're going to leave her so she can enjoy some alone time. Tell her that if she needs anything at all, to call out to you and you'll be there. This simple act of attentiveness will make her feel like a goddess.

Tell her that there is nothing she needs to do except give you a five-minute warning before she'd like to get out of the bath. Confiscate the towels and her bathrobe, so that when she does indicate she's ready to hop out, you can give the towels and robe a quick tumble dry to warm them for her.

After she's dried off in ultra-indulgent hot towels, and she's engulfed in a warm robe, lead her to the bed which has been turned down by you and has a chocolate waiting on the pillow for her. Bring her book to her to read in bed if she wishes, and give her feet a massage until she's ready to drift off into deep, much-desired sleep.

Extra Zing

To draw out your loving gift of time for her, extend it beyond just one evening. When she's out of the bath and relaxing in bed, kiss her and tell her there's more. Give her a card in which you've written how much you adore her and want to spoil her, along with four vouchers for indulgent pampering. These might be for a massage, body wrap, facial and manicure/pedicure. If you don't know her favorite beauty salon, you can buy these vouchers over the internet—just choose a place that looks luxurious and is convenient to your home, so it's not too difficult to arrange for her to get there. Tell her you've booked the sessions once a week for the next four weeks, and reassure her that you're going to take care of anything that needs doing in order to free up the time for her to take one hour a week for herself. Your thoughtfulness will make her feel every inch your beloved, and this gift of love will be one that keeps on giving—for you both.

Voyeur's Dream Cake

Watch me do me.

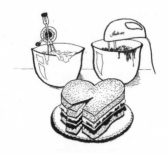

Pleasure Pantry Ingredients
His favorite pair of her sexy undies
Water-based lube or massage oil
Dish or saucer
Vibrator

Preparation
Watching your partner touch themselves sensually and sexually can be more arousing than even the most exotic porn. This is because the show is provided by your partner, and it's most definitely just for you, for your eyes only. And it's even better when you're both getting pleasure at the same time.

The key to mutual self-satisfaction here is to be mindful. Keep in the moment. Have a sexual encounter together purely focusing on your bodies. Give your full attention to every detail of how your body feels as you touch it, how your partner's body feels and responds to their own touch and also to yours. Don't drift off into a fantasy. Eagerly concentrate, and observe each other. Be attentive to the types of touch they give themselves: the rhythm, motions and pace.

Watch and learn—watch and *yearn*. Touch yourselves until you ache to touch each other.

Bring to Boil

Mutual pleasuring can be done in almost any setting, at any time, but can be fun to do in the daylight so you can really watch each other. It's a nice option for an afternoon delight, when the sun is warm and bathing both of your bodies in soft light.

Create a sacred space by sitting across from each other, and start with a simple Tantric breathing exercise. This will slow down your sexual response, increase your concentration on each other and strengthen the bond between you.

For the breathing exercises place your hands on each other's palms, sitting across from each other closely so your knees touch. Being close is important to connect you to each other, and to help you to breathe together. Start by breathing slowly in and out, initially holding each inhalation and exhalation for a count of four. Slowly start to elongate your exhalations to relax your bodies. Then each of you take one hand and place it over your partner's heart so you can feel their heartbeat, and help you to regulate your breathing rates until they are even and matched.

When you can't withstand the desire any longer, both of you move your other hand down to your nether regions. Slowly touch yourself to bring initial arousal. When you start to get really horny, start touching yourself with both hands.

If you're not already nude, take your undies off and spread your legs wide enough apart so you can get the best possible view of each other. One of you take the lube or oil and pour some in a dish or saucer, then place it between you.

Both of you can dip your fingers in it to grease your self-touch. Knowing that you're not touching each other (yet) but that you're linked by using and sharing the same lube at the same time can feel wildly different and strangely sexy.

Watch each other and quietly decide whether you want to mimic each other's tempo, or do what feels best for you, hoping the other will watch and mimic those motions on you later.

She can take her panties and reach over and wrap them around his dick. He can continue to masturbate, with his favorite undies of hers tightly coiled around the base of his cock. He can then take her favorite vibrator, dip it in the lube and lightly rub it up and down her lower lips. He can then take one of her hands and wrap it around the toy to get her to use it on herself. If it's a remote-controlled toy, he can keep the remote and surprise her by pressing the buttons to change speed and pressure.

Talk to each other, telling each other how much you like what you see—or say nothing at all. Look into each other's eyes, or gaze only at each other's, and your own, hands. Smile, laugh and show each other your enjoyment.

How intense you want to get is up to you. Experiment with touching each other, and then touching yourself again. Reach over and feel how hard he his. Take some of his lube or pre-cum and wipe it on yourself. Touch her pert clit and slide your hand down her inner lips, putting one or two fingers inside her and then rubbing her juice onto the head of your dick. If she comes first, she can keep stimulating herself for a second and third course until she comes again, simultaneously with his orgasm. If he comes first, he can watch her get off, seeing how she likes it.

The next day, before he leaves the house, she can surreptitiously hide those same panties either in one of his pockets or in his briefcase, to find later and remember the sight and touch of her. He can sneakily buy her a voice-activated sex toy and send it to her in the post, with a card that says, "Tell me next time you want to touch your sweet cake and I'll talk you through it, before eating you until your every desire is licked."

Extra Zing

Have a couple of races. Rule: absolutely no touching each other. Just watching while you touch yourself. For the first race, challenge each other to see who can come first. To keep it relatively fair, no toys allowed: just hands and lube. Start at the same time and rub vigorously until one of you comes first. It's easier to tell if the man comes first because he will (usually) ejaculate so, unless she's a female ejaculator, she's on trust to be completely honest and not fake an orgasm simply to win. There's no honour in a *faux* victory.

Your second race can have the opposite aim: to each stave off orgasm longer than the other. This is a bit like staring at each other to see who blinks first. The concentration and focus on what you're doing, yet forbidding climax for as long as possible, will make it even harder not to come. Both of you have to agree to the rule that you continuously touch yourselves—no cheating by taking pauses and lifting your hand away. The winner gets to make all the choices about your next sexual encounter: where, when, how. Wow.

your *pièce de (ir)résistance* by signing it. Most artists
[ha]ve their signature at the bottom, so reach down
[your] final word by signing your name, with your fin-
[ger o]r tongue, on their most private part.

[In] the experience of lust for each other, play a
[sex]y Scrabble together, using erotic words to spark
[your] imagination. First, each of you should separately
[list] what you'd like your partner to do for you if you
[win the ga]me, and put those desires in an envelope—no
[r]ule: it must be something sexy, and it can't
[be int]ercourse.

[Up the] ante of your sexy Scrabble game by making it Strip
[or Tea]n Strip Scrabble, all the words you are allowed to
[use are], teasing, passionate and dirty, and when you strike
[a le]tter your partner has to remove an item of clothing.
[If you] hit a triple letter score, your partner has to remove
[an item of] clothing and use the word in a saucy sentence to
[You'l]l be laughing and lusting in no time, so that no
[matter wh]o scores the highest, you both win.

Lust Letters

Letters of steaming lust for each other,
on each other.

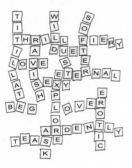

Pleasure Pantry Ingredients
Body paint and paintbrush
Wine (or similar)
Candles
Notepad
Marker pen
Scrabble (optional)
Paper and envelope (optional)

Preparation
When it comes to sex, the power of language can be hot.
Words stimulate our brain—our most important sexual
organ—whether they are said aloud, read, sent in a love
letter or written all over our bodies.

Prepare for this loving and demonstrative communication
with each other by first making sure that you have purchased
your ingredients. In most sex shops, even online, you can buy
a body paint set. These are edible paints in varying colors and
tastes. Body paints are usually washable, so they won't stain

your sheets, but you might want to check first—you wouldn't want anything to mar your enjoyment of the experience together.

Set up the bedroom beforehand with a bottle or carafe of wine, and light candles around the room. Entice your partner into the room by leaving a trail of one-word notes from the lounge to the bedroom. You can choose your own invitation, but it might look something like:

Come
Join
Me
For
Whatever
You
Want
As
Long
As
You
Want

Bring to Boil

When your lover arrives, pour them a glass of wine and give them a few shallow kisses, stimulating them lightly on their lips and tongue, where there are more sensitive nerve endings than deep in the mouth. Don't get too carried away, though—this session has only just started. (At this point you can choose to remove all your clothing, or only a bit. It depends on how you'd like to draw out your play.)

Take turns giving and receiving letters of lust. You might trace some letters and words along your partner's back and neck with just your finger first. Play with the curls and lines

of the letters, swoopi
shoulder blades, and
waist. You might write
ters only, and give ther
part by whispering to t
is for how beautiful yo
you. N is for the nape
touching. S is for sexy, v
with your words of lust
devote time entirely to o

If you want to have li
a serious seduction, play
most answers right wins
and gets to dictate where
drawn. Increase the sensat
game, by not only signing
but now also your tongue.

As you start to have fun
and begin painting your pa
the brush, think of their bo
ness as your muse, and expo
them with your adoring art
as you color in parts of them-
Adam's apple, or lips and eye
write words along their limb
want to use: tremble, urge, pu
fondle, touch, cock, pussy, wa
wish, delight, thrill, flicker, e
sweet, minx, vamp, vixen, wild
suck, lick, do, don't stop, right
softer, fuck, me, hot, you, incre

Finish off
and poets le
and have the
gers and yo

Extra Zing
To heighten
game of sex
your sexual
write down
win the ga
peeking!
include int

Up the
Scrabble. I
use are ho
a double le
When you
an item o
you. You'
matter wh

Dot Cum

The technology tease.

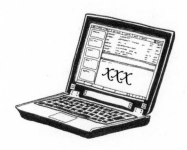

Pleasure Pantry Ingredients
Cell phone
Computer
Webcam (optional)

Preparation

Teasing your lovee from a distance is particularly thrilling because it lets them know that you're thinking about them, even when—and especially when—they're not near you.

Whether you're apart only for the day, or for longer, teasing through virtual technology can give you both a very real buzz. Connections made over the internet, or through text, can increase your lover's desire by giving them unambiguous hints of what's to come later. Many people find that they are better able to talk directly about what they want to do, or like having done to them, without face-to-face contact. If filthy talk isn't your forte, start with a flirty text ... and then work down to deliciously debauching yourselves with some dirty text.

Bring to Boil

Mobile phone texting is perfect for those short, sweet teasers to whet the sexual appetite. Use some of these tried and tested playful lines, or substitute them for some of your own as you discover the Joy of Text.

> Old bed. New trick.
> Can you work late tonight? I'm busy preparing. Myself. For You.
> Bedroom. 9 p.m. And not a minute sooner.
> Tonight you go first. And second. And third.
> Bought you something … but it needs double A batteries.
> Bring some home!
> Don't work too hard today—you'll need your energy for what
> I have in store for you tonight.
> One guess where my other hand is as I write this and think of
> you.
> Can you have too much? Let's find out!
> You're welcome, in advance.

After one, or a flurry, of flirty texts, you can escalate to longer, ruder passages through email. Send your lovee a graphic description of what you're going to do today:

> Driving to the store, I'm going to think of your dick inside me.
> Looking at the fruit and vegetables, I'm going to picture their
> moist, tender flesh and how good it will feel when you rub it
> all over my pussy, which is so hot right now I can feel every
> throbbing pulse as my lips get thick with want for you.

Or you might write them a wishful desire of what you want that night:

> As soon as I come in the door, you pull me to the bedroom. I
> don't have time to take my tie or shoes off. I don't even sit
> down. You unzip me and take my instantly hard dick in your
> mouth. You can't wait. You're on your knees. And when I come,
> you love it. You want more. And you'll get more. I'm cumming
> home at seven …

If you're both at the office, have a "Net nooner," engaging in
cybersex together on your lunch break. You can create a fantasy world of excitement by going a step further and
forming sexual cyberchick and cyberdick personas.

Open free email accounts using fake names that become
your saucy cyber identities. Make a date for a naughty nooner
through those accounts, but then rendezvous through an
instant messaging system so you can be more direct. With
your alternate identity, say things to your "new" partner that
you wouldn't dream about saying as yourself. But keep a firm
boundary around this other sexual personality, so that even if
your partner comments later about how hot that nooner was,
pretend not to know what they're talking about—"I don't
know any Juicy Jane. She sounds like a firecracker of a fantasy.
If you're having random erotic encounters on the internet,
that's very naughty." Give them a sly smile to indicate that you
want to keep your dot-cumming experiences separate, for
fun and filth, and then later send him an insistent must-meet-
again email from Juicy Jane.

Extra Zing

While the technology tease can be exciting enough, partially
because so much is left to the imagination, lots of men—and
women—like to upgrade their sexual hard drives by

watching. Dirty text and erotic emails can suffice for some, but others want more intensity to their internet interludes.

Webcam sex is rude, nude and in your face. Whether you or your lovee are into internet porn or not, redirect your sexual attention to watching each other and turning each other on, on screen. Strip for your partner, giving them peeks at you from the front, and behind. Let them watch you get off touching yourself. You can do this all in silence— restricting the sense of sound can sometimes intensify their response, because in their fantasy they can ignite a whole sultry script of what they want you to be thinking as they watch you. Or you can message them in real time to direct their self-touch and have them strip for you. The thrilling sense of feeling like you're controlling a partner's every sexual motion is a heady rush like no other.

Suite Show and Tell

Turn on bedtime reading to bedtime believing.

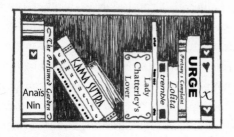

Pleasure Pantry Ingredients

Erotic fiction book(s)
Notepad and two pens
Costumes (optional)
Hotel room (optional)

Preparation

Fantasies can provide vital sexual energy release and allow for immense sexual creativity. While many men and women have private sexual fantasies and naughty thoughts which they would never want to act out in reality, actually fostering a few fantasies that you do want to enact as a couple can add a substantial serve of spice to a relationship, and a whole new erotic world to explore together.

To prepare, all you need to do is comb through a few good bookshops or online sex shops for some erotic books to share and read together.

Bring to Boil

Once you've bought an erotic book, put it on your bedside table. When the right night presents itself, reach over and start reading it aloud to your partner. Take turns reading passages to each other. You may find that the stories turn you both on so much that you fondle each other. You can bring each other to external orgasm (remember, this is a "Nibble night": an erotically pleasing evening, not a bonking session), or you can simply satisfy your arousal by listening and allowing yourself to flow with the words you hear and say. The passionate passages can lead you into a stirring dream time that you extend night after night, or can be a journey of erotic imaginings that fuel the fantasies you'd like to act out with each other. Tell each other when passages really turn you on, and reread them out loud for emphasis. Let your partner know when you read or hear elements of the erotic fantasies that you'd actually like to do and have done to you.

When you're quite rehearsed reading erotica written by others, try writing a fantasy of your own and leaving it somewhere unexpected for your lover to stumble upon. The more vivid it is, the better, because the wonderfully wicked devil is in the details. The graphic teasing builds sexual tension, and imagination, which heighten the pleasure when it arrives.

If you receive a surprise fantasy story written by your lovee, enhance the effect it has on you by asking them to read it to you, naked. Save it in your bedside drawer to use in times of self-pleasure, and to use as future foreplay. Every time you pull it out, the echo of its sexual lure will propel you right back to the powerful pleasure you experienced the very first time you read it, or heard it. This is pillow talk at its best because it turns a sexual monologue into a seductive dialogue between your bodies.

Extra Zing

To really take sharing a sexual fantasy to the next level, write one together and then act it out in every explicit detail. Prolong this experience by sharing it over several nights, at least. On the first night, lure your partner into the bedroom and sit together on the bed with a notepad and pens; tell them you're going to spark each other's sexual imagination by writing a fantasy together. Start with the first line and share your ideas one at a time, giving voice to both of your desires.

Since this fantasy is one you're going to act out, the details should be realistic for you. The realism will enhance the anticipation, because with each line you write, you know that one day soon it's all going to take place, right through to the happy ending. The first line can start with the practical:

They met at _____
[insert name of bar, park or other location]

Express every detail and then write:

His name was _____
[she fills in what name she'd like him to be]

Her name was _____
[he fills in what name he'd like her to be]

He was wearing _____
[she fills in what she'd like him to wear, including inner and outer clothing layers, and cologne]

She was wearing _____
[he fills in what he'd like her to wear, from her undergarments to the color of her clothes, and
nails to her perfume, the amount of make-up she has on, and how her hair is done.]

He was a _____
[she fills in what persona or profession she'd like him to have]

She was a _____
[he fills in what persona or profession he'd like her to have]

She was instantly attracted to him because _____

_____
[she writes how she wants him to behave at first]

And he was immediately turned on by her because _____

_____
[he writes how he wants her to behave]

When he talked to her he was _____

_____
[she writes what she'd like him to be when talking to her—
romantic, dirty, specific, courting, etc]

When she talked to him she was _____

_____
[he writes how he'd like to be spoken to—explicitly, seductively, romantically, earnestly, etc]

They flirted, kissed and touched each other's _____

_____
[she writes some parts of her body she'd like to have touched in public, and the places on
him she'd like to caress, and he writes the same from his desirous point of view]

Things get hot, so they decided to go to _____
[name hotel where they book a suite for the night]

Once in the suite, he _____
[she writes what she'd like him to do to her once inside the door. If she's shy writing this, she
can put it on a separate piece of paper to then show it her lover later]

60

And in the suite she _____

[he writes what he'd like her to do to him once inside the door. If preferred, he can do this separately and share it with her when they've both stopped writing]

End your written fantasy together with:

And this hot encounter happened on _____

[choose a date together and then book the hotel for that night, which may be in the next week or in two months' time. Then let the anticipation build as you both find yourselves fantasizing about this upcoming experience and how you can embody your partner's longings]

The details of a joint fantasy can require and stimulate a lot of thought, because it's thrilling to know it all may come true, and since you will both want to make the absolute most of this fantasy meeting and mating, feel free to take more than one evening as a Nibble night to write down your every will and wish, together or separately.

When you do come to act out your fantasy, you're both likely to get caught up in the heat of the moment, and that's why it's important to have your written tease serve as a general sexual essence guide rather than an exact script.

Once you do hit your date to act out your fantasy, maintain your personas throughout your entire night and morning in the suite, and then check out and go about your day separately. Meet each other back at home that next evening, and act as if nothing happened.

After a few days, leave your lover a note on the hotel stationery. Address it to their fantasy name, express your appreciation for that fantastic night, tell them you're going to be back in town in another couple of months—and invite them for another night together then.

To be continued . . .

Hot

*W*arm
like fire,
permanent
like ink in skin,
smooth
like good brandy,
you go down well.

The Cat's Meow

Make her purrrrr with your touch and technique.

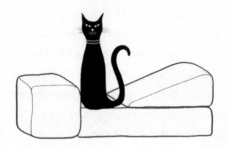

Pleasure Pantry Ingredients
Pillows
Liberator

Preparation

The beauty of finding a new technique for a position that can enhance both his and her pleasure is that no preparation is needed except to learn how to do it. The Coital Alignment Technique (CAT) is a variation of the man-on-top position and so can be substituted for the classic man-on-top (missionary) position whenever you both feel you would like to maximize the experience of orgasm during intercourse. This may be on usual nights of sex, or on special occasions when you feel like putting in a bit of new effort and creativity.

According to international research, less than 30 percent of women are able to reliably come during penile-vaginal intercourse. This research reflects a simple anatomical fact: women are simply not designed for maximum pleasure through penetration. If they were, the vagina would be rich with pleasurable nerve endings, enabling the penis thrusting in and out to easily deliver her to ecstasy. But if this really were the case, and the vagina really did have a vast network of nerves that respond to stimulation, simple activities like the insertion of tampons, fingers, speculums—even experiences such as Pap smears and childbirth—would be orgasmic. And, of course, we know they are not. So why would we think that the penis, as fantastic as it may be, would suddenly transform this vaginal canal into an orgasmic space if nothing else can?

The truth is that there are very few pleasing nerve endings in the vagina. The central area of female sexual nerve endings is in the clitoris (8000 of them alone in the glans!), the inner and outer lips, the perineum—the stretch of skin between the vaginal opening and the anus—and at the entrance of the vagina. So, while she does experience *pleasure* through penetration—and especially enjoys stimulation right at the entrance of her vagina—she mostly, and primarily, experiences *sexual pleasure* all along the outside, sliding from her clitoris down towards the entrance of her vagina. The CAT is designed to maximize this whole outer area, rather than the deep inner vagina, during intercourse, to bring both her and him to orgasm—sometimes even together.

Bring to Boil

The Coital Alignment Technique is a favorite among couples who like to make love face to face, bodies connected, and with both partners given equal opportunity to come. As it's a variation of the man-on-top position, the CAT requires the man to do a few things differently, and the variations are critical for her pleasure.

One difference is that he rests his body weight on her, or to the side of her, rather than on his arms or elbows. When the man has to support his own weight he tends to come faster, and one of the requirements for coming together—or at least both coming during intercourse—is to last longer, to give the woman enough time to reach orgasm. Next, the man "rides high"—that is, he shifts himself up so that when he is inside her, the base of his penis is in contact with her clitoris. However, deep thrusting is not the aim of this game; instead, both partners engage in rocking and rubbing motions so that, as his penis continues to receive stimulation, contact with her clitoris is never interrupted. This is the key ingredient to pussy-friendly CAT loving: do not break cock-base-to-love-button friction! As they grind and rock, he keeps contact through his downward-into-her motion, and she keeps the pressure on with her up-against-him rocking. To alternate sensation she can wrap her legs around him, resting her ankles on his calves for a slightly deeper penetration while still maintaining ideal pelvic contact, or she can straighten her legs out directly under his for a very shallow penetration that increases the rubbing along her clitoris.

For added variety, and if increased shaft stimulation is needed for him to reach high arousal, partners can alternate positions to her on top for a few minutes. This will allow much deeper penetration and stimulation for him, while still enabling direct access to her clitoris. She may even orgasm while on top, and this will only enhance her ability to come again once back in the man-on-top CAT position. The clitoris becomes erect (just like the penis) so once she's experienced an orgasm, the glans of her clitoris will be fully engorged with blood and even more alert and responsive to the stimulation from the base of his penis during the final grinding in the CAT position.

To enhance the CAT position for an even more intense bodily effect, place a pillow under her lower back to create a pelvic tilt upwards towards his groin. She'll be positively purring with delight at the experience of not just one but two or more orgasms during intercourse!

Extra Zing

To bring the Kama Sutra to life in a multitude of purrfectly pleasurable positions for you both, try using "sexational" furniture such as the Liberator Bedroom Adventure Gear. Liberator Shapes (available to order online) is a set of five sex-enhancement pieces, designed to be put together a variety of ways for both partners to experience greater pleasure and comfort while experimenting with a number of positions. A flat bed will feel ever so mundanely horizontal once you've tried sex on the Liberator furniture.

The CAT technique can be enhanced using the pieces by adding a wedge underneath her to create a further pelvic tilt so that his pelvis has even greater contact with hers, and to give her an upward angle that allows more access to the clitoris, while also enabling deeper penetration during the position. Once you've stimulated both her clitoris and his shaft with the CAT on the sexational pieces, increase the wedges behind her back so that she is better able to lean up and forward under him, while still having her back supported. You can take this even further to a fully supported sitting position.

The CAT is about finding the right angle, and using pillows or something like Loving Angles can get you both loving the sensation, support and, yes, the pivotal pelvic angle. Twist yourselves into an intertwined incline that will give you a whole new slant on mutual pleasure!

Rockin' Roll

Live and love by the roll of the dice.

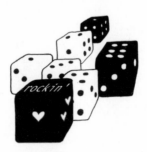

Pleasure Pantry Ingredients
"Love dice"
Red or black bed sheets
Red light bulbs—2
Standard dice—5 sets
Fluffy dice
His and hers matching robes (optional)
Evening beverage of choice (whiskey optional)
Hotel or cabin for the weekend (optional)

Preparation
One of the primary sexual issues which couples face after a while is "routine" sex—the thrill of unpredictable passion can wane when couples have made love hundreds or thousands of times over the years. To put a bit of unpredictable anticipation and sexual curiosity back into the bedroom, roll the dice ... and see what comes up.

To prepare, you need to obtain at least one set of "love dice." These can be purchased through a sex shop (online or bricks and mortar) or even through a joke shop. There are a few different versions of love dice but typically they are a set of dice (some glow in the dark for between-the-sheets play) in which one die indicates "what to do" while the other die shows "where to do it." This might be where on the body, or where in the house!

Buy your partner and yourself matching robes. If you can, find polka dot robes to maximize the theme of the night. Or else, enhance the roll-of-the-dice/love-gambling theme by getting robes in sexy roulette black or red. Slip a set of the love dice in the pocket of their robe and hang both your robes in your bedroom, bathroom or dressing room/wardrobe.

While it's optional to buy or even just wear robes, purchasing a new set of sexy bedroom gear for you both can add a sense of novelty and excitement. If you build a theme by making up your bed with new red or black sheets and placing red light bulbs in your bedside lamps, with both of you wearing new robes to remove from each other, and you start rolling the dice in this sexy atmosphere, the effort you go to will help both of you embrace this new gambling, spontaneous lovemaking, and make the most of your love game. Sex is a sensual activity, and an imaginative setting can create just the right mood for a roll . . .

Bring to Boil

Once you've set up the bedroom, with red light bulbs in your bedside table lamps and red or black sheets on the bed, turned down, put on your robe and flirtatiously invite your partner to put on their own robe. As they do, prepare a drink for each of you to sip as you start to play. This can be a beverage of your choice, but you may like to continue with the sexual gambling theme by pouring a gambler's drink of whiskey. If not, choose wine—or a nonalcoholic drink, to keep your stamina up!

Once you return to the bedroom, join your partner on the bed and invite them to feel in their robe pocket (if they haven't already done so) to discover the dice.

Take turns rolling the dice and obeying the rules of each toss. If your love dice direct you to do certain saucy things in other rooms in the house, you must do so! If you risk being caught by someone hearing you or walking in on you, be careful—but this danger can also heighten the thrill of the gamble.

After satiating yourselves with love play in turns and together, roll a pair of standard dice to gamble on when you might play with the love dice next—one die indicating which month for the next six months, and the other nominating the week. For example, if you roll 3 and a 2, your next Rockin' Roll night would be three months from now, in the second week of the month. Choose a night and mark your calendar!

To keep the game alive, and as a teasing reminder, take four sets of standard dice and hide them around the house for your lovee to find. You might leave dice in their work bag, gym bag, cosmetic drawer, kitchen utensil drawer, resting on a stack of books in the study . . . any unexpected place to give your lovee a reminder of the fun that sexual spontaneity can bring.

Or, for a constant reminder, hang a set of fluffy dice in their car, so they never forget that, while your relationship is a sure bet, your sex can be a fun gamble with only a roll of the dice!

Extra Zing

For a bit of extra oomph in your sexual game-playing, personalize the love dice game with your own rules. Choose a pair of mismatched standard dice so you can tell them apart (by color or size) and make a set of rules you both agree to play by. You might like to arrange the rules of the game that night, or on a preceding night to heighten the anticipation.

If you really want to add intensity to your new sexy spontaneity, choose a weekend to go away together. In the preceding weeks, roll the dice to decide who will arrange what. The first to roll a double has to take care of arranging the location and accommodation. And the first person to roll a six must take care of the necessities to get away (pet sitters, children's sleepovers, babysitters, etc). Once the arrangements have been made and you're ready to get away, ensure that you take your dice and your rules for your dirty weekend roll between the sheets. One die (a red one, for example) can be set for body parts, while the other one (perhaps white) can relate to specific sexual teases and kisses. The beauty of this game is that you can tailor it to the exact things you and your partner love to drive each other wild with.

Below are some sample ideas, but you can design your own spicy substitutions.

Sample rules:

Red die	White die
1 = mouth	1 = lick
2 = back	2 = stroke lightly
3 = inner thighs	3 = nibble
4 = neck	4 = blow hot breath
5 = butt	5 = tickle
6 = genitals	6 = tongue kiss

If someone rolls a double of anything, it can be seen as a "wild roll" and they can either take that option or choose any other thing they'd like their partner to do to them by simply requesting it as their double-roll "wild option." If someone rolls a double 1, they must reveal a sexual fantasy to the other. Last rule: a double 6 has no time limit!

Spend the weekend away together living and loving by the roll of the dice, thus infusing your romantic relationship with unpredictability and spontaneity by leaving all decisions to chance. Play together and make up your own rules; have fun by keeping your romantic relationship constantly on the edge of curiosity and unpredictability by betting with each other and living by fate and whim. Stay in or go out? Roll for it. Make love or eat? Roll for it. Take a drive or a walk? Roll for it. Have a quickie or a longer session? Roll for it! Then *go* for it!

From Here to There

Beach blanket bonking

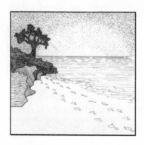

Pleasure Pantry Ingredients
Beach blanket or large towel
Skirt and G-string or sarong and bikini for her
"Easy access" shorts for him

Preparation

One of the most favorite locations for alfresco sex is the beach. "Sex on the beach" is so well known and desired, it's even a flirtatious cocktail! However, many who want to have beach sex often never try it, or don't end up going all the way because of the lack of privacy—or too much sand—while others who do manage the beach bonk spend an hour afterwards getting sand out of numerous bodily crevices.

The romance of beach seduction was, for many, immortalized in the famous scene in the 1953 film *From Here to Eternity*: Burt Lancaster and Deborah Kerr created an unforgettable image of two lovers swept up in the wild abandon of passion as they kissed at the edge of the surf, with the waves breaking over them, mimicking their crescendo of pleasure and desire.

That's Hollywood for you, though: an unrealistic image. Think, in reality, how impractical and uncomfortable that would be, especially if lust were to take over in that particular location! No: optimal beach sex isn't at the edge of the sea with the waves washing piles of sand up swimsuits. It's discreetly coveting each other's bodies while enjoying the view and experiencing the excitement of getting naturally sexual with each other in one of nature's most romantic and sexy locations.

Perfect beach sex is all about practical beach sex. Sand is an ingredient, but not the main staple—it doesn't go in everything! It is possible to have a fantastic, sand-free, fun-filled sexual beach frolic with just a little preparation and careful positioning.

Bring to Boil

Sex at the beach is often spontaneous and can be enjoyed in broad daylight, feeling the warmth of the sun on skin; at sunset or twilight after a lovely walk together; or at night, under the cover of darkness. Whenever it's done, though, the beach has two primary ingredients: water and sand. These don't have to play a role in optimal beach sex, though.

Spread out your blanket or towel and lie down on it to kiss and canoodle. Obviously, because sex in public view of anyone is illegal, it's important to choose a location that is secluded. This may be on a stretch of beach where no one else is around, or inland away from the surf, towards the dunes or brush. The best position is her on top, wearing a skirt or sarong. He should pull down his board shorts, Speedos or pants to his upper or mid-thigh—just low enough to provide access, but within reach of his arms to pull them up quickly should someone else come along. She can then remove her bikini bottoms, or slide her G-string off, or even just pull her clothing to one side. She can then straddle him, spreading out her skirt as she spreads her legs. A skirt or sarong automatically creates a covering so that if someone does walk by they won't be sure what's going on: whether it's simply a make-out session or actual sex. Under a skirt her bottom won't be exposed as she rides up and down on his shaft. As she's sitting on him she can grind her hips forwards and backwards, as well as pumping hard and fast on top of him, knowing all the while that, as wild as it gets, it's still discreet.

Ideal beach sex, for many, means indulging in the sensual location of the beach without experiencing the *specifics* of the beach—namely, sand in unwelcome places. This is made easier if both partners are dry rather than wet. Ocean water is salty and can create a sticky and slightly abrasive feeling on the skin as the lovers rub up and down each other. Wet skin also attracts caked-on sand. Some couples may prefer optimal beach sex when they are both dry—either after sunning themselves post-swim, or in the evening or night, without a swim. Dry skin allows sand to be simply brushed off hands, knees and back.

If, however, you do find yourselves engaging in the heat of the moment wet all over, release yourselves to the spontaneity of the moment, knowing that the towel under him and skirt or sarong over her will protect your private genital contact from sand, and then you can freely enjoy the salty feel of your partner's skin massaging and exfoliating your own. When you're both happy, feeling complete pleasure, he can reach under her skirt or through the slip of her sarong to finger her to a first, second or third orgasm, and then, as easily as you got into the discreet position, you can unfurl yourselves, stand up, immediately dressed as if you've been up to nothing at all, and continue your lover-ly beach swim or walk.

Beach sex may not get you from here to eternity, but it will get you from here to there—yes, yes, right, mmmm, there.

Extra Zing

For a bit of extra sizzle, have sex in the surf with the swell of the waves washing over you both. To experience optimal sex in water, it's best if you make out first in the water, arousing each other, until he has a hard erection. The water can wash away much of her natural lubricant, making entry more difficult, so it's best for him to stimulate her first and then penetrate her in one thrust if he can, to minimize the amount of water that may enter her vagina. If she removes her bikini bottoms and he lines up the head of his penis to the entrance of her vagina, then with one move enters her, it can be the most amazing experience of sex as both your weights are supported, allowing for a position many couples find difficult: standing with her wrapped around him. She can straddle his waist or hips with her legs to help stay connected, and he'll find it easiest to thrust and grind if he can still stand, rather than both treading water. Reach down (him or her) and rub her clitoris to enhance her arousal. The combination of weightless sex with the novelty of doing it in the ocean can make for exciting intercourse that can last as long, or as little, as you both like. Let the waves of ecstasy roll over you.

The 3 a.m. Special

Dreams do come . . . true.

Pleasure Pantry Ingredients
Alarm clock (vibrating preferred)
Pen and paper (optional)

Preparation
Middle-of-the-night sex rates as one of his top desires, so make it a reality he can really remember! Men experience a semi or hard rev of their sexual response approximately every 90 minutes, culminating in the ultra-hard Morning Glory erection—so middle-of-the-night sex is not only erotic for him as his fantasy becomes reality, but will take advantage of his growing arousal throughout the night.

As this sex scenario takes place in the middle of the night, there is no preparation required except to take measures to make sure you wake up in the small hours.

The sexual response—like every other part of our bodies—requires sleep to rejuvenate so, to maximize this erotic encounter, it's best to wait until the morning hours, well past midnight. While testosterone increases towards dawn, a time such as 3 a.m. allows at least four hours of pre-sex rest time (provided you both went to bed around 11 p.m.) and can then give your partner, and you, at least another two or three hours of sleep afterwards. So, even with such a delightful sleep interruption, no or little negative impact is felt the next day in terms of fatigue. Also, 3 a.m. is a time when you're likely to find your partner in a dreamy state of sleep; waking them will be a slow process, and one in which you can gently eroticise their dream state before they realize that their erotic dream isn't a dream after all but actually, really, happening to them ...

To prepare, make sure you pick a night when the next day is like any other—don't pick a night before a big meeting or deadline. Make sure your timing is such that it's a complete surprise for him, and a night when it will be met with pleasure, not stress.

Set an alarm clock before you go to bed. Because you will want to wake him with your touch, try to use a quiet, vibrating alarm tucked under your pillow, or on your side of the bed, rather than a noisy alarm that will also wake him when it sounds.

Bring to Boil

Once the alarm goes off, take a moment to wake up and turn on—but don't wake up completely, because you too can enjoy the sensation of half-dreamy eroticism by rolling over to your partner and spooning into him, creating body heat between you to remind you why you set your alarm, and why you're surprising your man with a 3 a.m. Special.

With your eyes closed, or half open, transition from sleep to awake by stroking your hand up and down the length of your body, and your partner's body. Start to concentrate on his nether region, caressing his thighs and hips.

Nudge your head under the sheets and take his dick in your mouth. Don't strip the sheets down for access, because you want to make his transition from sleep to semi-awake slow, and if you expose his whole body to the fresh air he might either wake up or turn over, or even try to pull the sheets back up over him.

Nestle down in the bed with your face kissing and licking his shaft, head and balls. As he begins to become erect, become more insistent with your mouth, giving him firm oral pleasure, and cup his balls in your hand to create heat and sensation there. If he wakes up enough to respond to you verbally, or try to take control by pulling you over so he can penetrate you (not an uncommon response because, once aroused, especially from sleep, he'll likely be on autopilot to get to orgasm and want to take control to get there), push him back down and whisper to him, "*Sshhh*. It's the middle of the night and you're having a wet dream from me. Lie back and enjoy."

Continue kissing his thighs up to his hip bones, lower belly, navel, and back down on his dick. Don't spend any time above his navel, unless it's to reach up and massage his chest and arms with your hands. If you raise your head above the sheets and engage in face-to-face contact it can break his dreamlike state, as he might be tempted to open his eyes and connect with you, then want to dominate the experience as he wakes. If you stay concentrated on his lower regions he's more likely to keep his eyes closed and remain in a semi-sleepy state, while part of his brain takes in the physical stimulation you're giving him and the other part gets hijacked by erotic thoughts of you, and of sex.

When his dick is throbbing with desire and heat, climb on top of him—making sure to keep the sheets over you both (unless it's a sweltering hot night)—and guide his cock inside you. Because this is night-time sleepy sex, start with slow, rhythmic movements, grinding your hips, through your lower back, backwards and forwards. Lean forward and give him hot mouth kisses on his neck. Let him relax totally in the dark and simply receive. Don't motion or ask for him to do anything.

As you ever so slowly rock your hips on him, front and back, side to side and up and down, with his dick inside you, lower one hand and rub your clitoris, allowing yourself to move with him inside you to your personal sexily selfish rhythm as you touch yourself to orgasm. Try not to have a screaming orgasm but a melting one that's quieter, to keep the dreamlike ambience.

Once you've come, prop your body weight so you can bounce on him until you bring him to orgasm. Many men may really enjoy a slow, seductive start, especially if they've been asleep for the first part of the arousal, but to come home they often like a hard and furiously fast finish. Give him this relief to release by spreading out your hands to the side of his shoulders so you can brace your upper body, and pulse your pelvis up and down the whole length of his shaft until he comes. He likely became highly aroused while you had an orgasm on top of him so, to bring him to his climax an even and very fervent pace up and down his shaft will get him there in no time.

Once he's come, lean down and kiss his neck and cheek. Don't engage his mouth—let him simply be touched without ever having to respond. Allow him to be the total recipient of your touch and desire. Then roll off and lie next to him, spent and ready for sleep again, letting your breathing become even until you're both asleep again. No pillow talk, no romantic expectations—simply a middle-of-the-night special surprise: nocturnal nookie.

Extra Zing

If you want to extend the experience of the 3 a.m. Special for you both, get up afterwards and write a description of the sex you had together, then leave it for him to find somewhere the next day. Make your description of the sex very detailed, writing exactly what you did to him and why, including the sensations you felt and why you enjoyed them. Especially because this is an experience you controlled from start to finish, it's an excellent way to communicate to him what you like and why.

Write the whole experience as if it were a dream. Start your description with "I had the most amazing dream last night . . . I woke up and I was so turned on by your sleeping body that I then . . ." and after your description end it with "Was it a dream or real? Did you have it too? Did you like it too?"

Tit for Tat

Brand her yours . . .

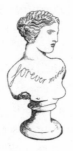

Pleasure Pantry Ingredients
Lipstick
Temporary tattoo stickers
Henna ink and drawing pen
Water-based ink markers
Shaving cream (optional)
Razor (optional)

Preparation
In an equal relationship—which is what many couples strive for—a balance is sought: in domestic duties and co-parenting, in work and investment in the home, family and relationship, and in expressing desire and affection for the other. "What I give you, you give me; what I do for you, you do for me" might sound like balance, but sometimes a relationship, especially a sexual one, isn't so easily measured out that evenly. An equal relationship, sexually, is one in which both partners feel satisfied and happy, desired and connected. The idea that an equal, balanced sex life means that both partners initiate sex equally, take spicy risks equally, and romance

equally, is great in theory but not always practiced. Sometimes, for a woman to feel hot, desired and intensely sexual, she doesn't want equality—she simply wants to be possessed. This is a very non-"PC" approach to sex, but sex isn't always a political expression of equality and division of labor in a relationship. Sometimes sex is about raw desire, and nothing greater.

One of the most common fantasies many women have is to be taken by a stranger, ravished without complete consent, and possessed totally by another because she is so incredibly irresistible. This "you must be mine" is *fantasy only*—in no way does it mean that a woman wants to be taken against her will in actuality, nor is it a justification for relationship, date or stranger rape, which are absolutely wrong and against the law. But within the boundaries of a mutually affectionate, consensual relationship, the thrill of being desired so intensely that your lover wants to mark you as his own can bring a heat of want in a woman unlike anything else. Change the sexual pace for once, from equitable partner to branded woman, and set the sparks flying.

Prepare by obtaining some cheap lipstick from the drugstore so you can brand her in red. Also, most drugstores or natural health stores will have henna, or mehendi, for dying hair and skin (many Indian women have their hands and feet decorated with intricate designs with this, and modern temporary "henna tattoos" have become popular). If you don't want to go for henna, which can last for well over a week or more, you can get some water-based ink pens or markers which will often last just a few days, and that might be long enough for you both. Once you have your ingredients, think about the kinds of designs and phrases you want to brand your partner with. Prepare some hot talk to turn her on as you mark her.

Couples who tattoo themselves with each other's names or initials do this because they want a permanent etching as testament to their love. Mark your lover in this same way, while telling her the whole time what you feel and what you're writing. The henna or ink tattoos aren't permanent like a real tattoo, but the imprint of your love and desire will be everlasting.

Bring to Boil

Invite your lovee into the bedroom and ask her to lie down on her front so you can give her a skin massage. Rather than give her a deep-muscle massage, tell her you're going to relieve and invigorate her largest organ: her skin. Trace your fingers ever so lightly from the base of her neck, along her back, up and down in long, relaxing strokes. Let your hands travel from her back across the roundness of her butt cheeks, and down along her thighs, calves and ankles. Create a slow, long rhythm, moving your hands lightly all the way up and all the way down her body. Move to her arms, tracing your fingers up from her wrists to her neck and onto the side of her face. Swirl your fingers gently along her jaw line, cheeks, temples and eyelids.

Tell her how much you love her. Tell her what about her body you love, and why. Women are auditory: they fall in love and stay in love based largely on what they hear from their partner. It's important, as a man, to not only appreciate her visually, and also through deeds, but to tell her over and over why she is so special to you, what about her turns you on, why you love her and love being her lover. As you express all this to her, tell her that you're going to make her yours, all over. That you want to make her body a canvas dedicated to how much you love her, and how you want to worship every inch of her as if she were a temple to your feelings.

Start with the lipstick, and draw on her upper arm. Because the permanent ink will stay for at least a few days, it's best to use lipstick, which is relatively easily washed away, on parts of her body that may be seen in public. As hot as you are now, together in bed, she's the one who might have to do the shopping or front up at the office with "I want to touch your body all the time" written up her arm— and that might not be so sexy in that setting, so best to keep the permanent ink for the private words in private places.

Using the lipstick, henna dye or marking pens, express all your inner desires to her by writing them down on her body. Remember, this is a game of feelings, not equitable politics, so write what you feel. You might write things like "You're mine, all mine," "Property of ..." or "Only I touch here," drawing an arrow to an intimate part of your lover's body. Draw circles around her nipples and love hearts on her butt cheeks, or write the dates of your first dinner, your first kiss, the first time you made love or your wedding all around her front. Pick a favorite love poem and write it along her back. Come up with a list of sexy adjectives to describe her and write them all along her legs. With so much pressure on women to look physically perfect and desirable, even the trimmest, tautest woman can suffer from body anxieties, so to have her lover write beautiful, sexy words on her, nude, is affirming to her that you do adore and desire her, and that she is incredibly sexy and the most beautiful woman to you. This can be a very powerful and erotic activity for both of you, and especially for her.

Make your last markings at the top of her inner thigh, high up into the crease near her outer sexual lips, slowly writing your first initial so she can look down and see it on her left side, and your second initial on the right side. With her branded all over, right down to her sexiest sacred area, kiss her, tell her you have to possess all of her now, push her down and insistently make love to her without pausing for breath. Talk to her as you thrust in and out of her, tell her everything you've ever wanted to say, everything you've ever felt about her as your lover. You've been expressing these feelings to her all evening, so continue with your words and feelings to a climactic crescendo. Telling her what you want to say in an experience like this will sear your words into her mind for ever; your passionate brand which will burn brightly in her long after the ink you've marked on her has faded.

When you're both satiated, write the day's date on her breast with the word "mine." Then write the day's date on the back of her hand. It will be visible to everyone, but it will be private code. And if someone asks her what the numbers on her hand means, tell her to say, "Just a reminder of something not to forget . . . "—code for "marked mine, branded for love."

Extra Zing

For an extra-sexy branding, leave the ink behind and take a razor instead. Undress your lover, then gently shave her pubic hair into a design of your choice. You may like to shave her completely bare, or leave a landing strip or small patch, or you may like to get creative and draw a heart or lightning bolt; or even your initials, if you have a good razor and enough time to devote to this activity.

Whatever you do, the eroticism is in the shaving, not the resulting design. She puts herself in a position of vulnerable trust, legs akimbo, with the razor in your hands, about to shave the hair of some of her body's most sensitive parts.

Smear on some shaving cream and lather it up, taking an effort to please her while you're there, to relax her as much as arouse her. Gently and slowly shave her from the triangle of hair at the top of her mound, down over her lips. Do this in front of a mirror, in the bathroom or with a hand-held mirror in the bedroom, so you can both watch the blade reveal her soft nakedness. When you're done, admire your work with an appreciative—very generously appreciative—touch on her. Tit for tat: she shaves you next!

Jazz Fever

Make beautiful music together.

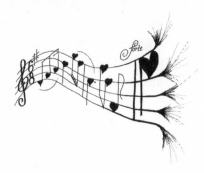

Pleasure Pantry Ingredients
Tickets to a jazz concert or invitation to a jazz bar
Jazz CD(s) on stereo

Preparation
If you associate music with making love, jazz would have to be at or near the top of the list for creative, erotic, sexy experimentation together. After all, a study from the National Opinion Research Center in Chicago found that jazz listeners had the most sex. With its ability to seductively sway as well as sweatily swing, much of jazz, whether it's improvisational or orchestrated, is like sex: communication between mouths, instruments and souls.

Bring to Boil
To get in the mood for a jazzy evening, head out to a jive bar before you dive between the sheets. Invite your partner to dress up and spend an evening of sexy music and company with you before you conduct your horizontal love session.

Both women and men love to dress up from time to time and see their lovee looking fabulously sexy, and since you'll both be dancing this is a perfect opportunity for him to don a suit or tux, and for her to wear a dress that flares on twirling and don dancin' heels. She can continue to get in the mood by channelling a feeling of "sultry" and he can channel feeling "masterful."

Step out on the town looking every inch the lovely, and in love, couple you are. Dancing is a sexy and enticing expression of the two of you in rhythm together, so spend an evening bending and arching into each other's bodies to create heat between you and a mutual tempo all your own. Notice how your bodies fit and how you communicate subtly yet so very clearly, without saying a word. When you want to switch your dancing from vertical to horizontal, head back to your place and let your shoulders and hips continue to sing of sex all the way home.

When it comes to mixing it up in your sex life, it's interesting to know that most couples have sex in one or two positions in any one session. While they may rotate the number of positions they use over time, many couples engage in limited position variety in any one sex session. To really get feverishly hot with lovemaking, put on your favorite jazz CD and make love like jazz musicians jam: with improvisation, solo instrument focus that explodes with energy, and lots of movements and combinations.

Start your sexual improvisation between the sheets by whispering sweet everythings to each other as you undress one another. Sing to your lovee, kiss them all over, and then concentrate on your lower-love-zone kissing. Ladies: skin-flute him by pulling your lips slightly apart, as if you were going to blow into a flute, and then exhale hot breath on him before softly flicking your tongue forwards and backwards across the tip of his head. Then lick and suck his instrument of pleasure with wide, firm lips to make him tremble and moan with desire. Gentlemen: blow her like a trumpet. Place the front of your lips so they rest gently against her clitoris, taking the tip in the soft, wet part of your inner lips. Purse your lips tight around her love button and nuzzle your lips while flicking the very tip of your tongue from side to side against her glans until she's quivering. Don't break your mouth seal on her until you can tell she wants even more heat, and even more intense, harder touch.

When it's time for an entangled tango together, remember that even the slightest variation can transform the way a position feels. Start with the man-on-top position, then vary it by swinging her legs over his shoulders, and then after a few thrusts stretch one of her legs up straight and gain entry from a diagonal hip-to-hip join. From here she can shift both her legs over to one side to create a slight twist, and tighter feel, in her vagina and along his shaft. Shift all the way over to a side-by-side position, spooning first, then, when you both want greater physical intensity, pull forward together onto your knees and go cheeky style (another name for doggy style—because you'll feel a bit cheeky doing it!) until she wants more control. She can push him onto his back and straddle him, riding him face to face. Then she can lie down on his chest, so body-on-body contact creates warmth and sensation from tip to toe.

Finish side by side, facing each other, mingling your sweat together. Look into each other's eyes and smile. Open-eyed sex can be very intimate; an open-eyed orgasm can be even more intimate. Don't throw your head back in solo ecstasy at climax: look your partner directly in the eyes as you come. Share your twitching, trilling, quavering response. It's fervent. It's feverish.

Extra Zing

Dance together after sex, naked. Wrap a blanket around the two of you and head outside, under the stars, for a moonlight waltz. Nights like these create beautiful memories to cherish for always. Live the love song.

Bush Tucker

Have a shag, then grab your swag! (Doing it Down Under, Aussie-style)

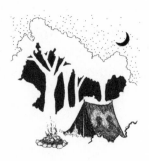

Pleasure Pantry Ingredients
Camping gear
Foam mattress
Tent
Fishing gear (optional)
Cowboy hat
G-string
Hiking boots/outdoor boots/ugg boots
Coffee
Rum
Whipped cream
Sleeping bag(s)
Thick blanket

Preparation

When it comes to romance, most people think of the traditional model of the man courting the woman with poems, chocolates, flowers and other tokens and demonstrations of his affection. Some women, on the other hand, are hardpressed to articulate how they romance their men. "I say yes to sex!" a few have jokingly said. But what is romance if not simple and genuine gestures of heartfelt desires and feelings? And how is this not absolutely 100 percent H-O-T? Presents aren't necessary for this kind of hot romance. In fact, in most harried couples' lives today, the gift of quality alone time together, away from mobile phone reception, computers, internet cafés, digital diaries, demanding children, robotic schedules and haranguing stress can be utterly priceless. It can also be highly rejuvenating to your relationship as can't-keep-my-hands-off-you lovers, in addition to the juggle of being partners, parents, peacemakers, moderators, caregivers and career moguls.

Now, if some people could choose anywhere to go to be alone together, camping outdoors in the full *au naturel* experience of nature would be the last place on earth. These are the type of people who don't like to "rough it." But for this dirty weekend in the bush, rough it together anyway, as an adventure.

Spend some quality time as a couple, doing some of what you do indoors in the great outdoors . . . and have fun doing it!

If you're already regular campers, or non-urban people, take this opportunity to have a sexy good time alone in the bush, without friends along or without having to work on the land. If, however, you're a camping virgin, look upon the weekend as a wild escapade. And if you know you hate camping but it's a favorite pastime of your partner's, going along and roughing it with them is the epitome of a wonderfully romantic gesture.

Prepare by choosing your location and getting all your camping gear packed and ready to go. A visit to a camping store will show you that roughing it doesn't have to mean going without much. Yes, you can opt for the luxury bush getaway, or you can get back to basics. With the latter, pack a billy can and loose tea. Otherwise, go ahead and purchase the takeaway espresso doo-hickey to make your must-have Italian coffee over the campfire. This sexy getaway is, after all, about seduction, not sacrifice.

As this is a romantic, rough-and-ready, sex-in-the-bush weekend outdoors, a little bit of comfort insurance is necessary for a truly good time. If you can, take a foam mattress. A double mattress that rolls up can easily fit in most two-man tents, or it can be used as extra padding under a swag (sleeping bag) by the campfire. Wonderful memories of lovemaking might not be generated if all you can remember is rocky terrain, grazed knees, sharp objects in the middle of your backs, and both of you grumpy because neither of you got any sleep! So an investment in a little bit of added padding is a sensible one. And to add extra entertainment to the camping erotica, make sure the whipped cream and G-string are hidden away as surprise sexy elements for him come darkness.

Bring to Boil

If at all possible, drive to a place where you can set up camp alone rather than to a caravan park or camping ground. If you have no choice about how isolated you can get, try to choose your camping weekend away at a time that isn't high season, so you can find a little patch of bush to yourselves.

Before you christen the tent, engage in fresh outdoor activities together. Get your blood pumping and enjoy your alone time together. If there's a fishing spot nearby, sit together and enjoy your surroundings as you fish. Enjoy the fact that there are limited distractions, especially of the electronic variety, and embrace this time to talk together, about anything, about everything.

If you can find a place to be completely alone, encourage your partner to join you in a skinny dip in a creek or river. Throw yourselves over to wild abandon—be flirtatiously feral together! Get back to nature ... all the way.

Once back at your camp site, if you have some privacy you might like to tease your man by strutting around in little more than your birthday suit. Pop a cowboy hat on your head, strip out of your clothes down to your G-string and boots (in colder temperatures, wear knee-high ugg boots and a coat) and go about the business of getting dinner ready at camp. Most people associate camping with being wrapped up in bulky, unsexy clothes, so toss the stereotype away and embrace raw, natural sexuality as you wiggle your bottom all around him. You'll be a visual magnet for him—even if you're in a place with stunning views, his eyes will follow only you.

Once you've munched down on your bush tucker, cooked over the campfire (very ruggedly romantic!), ask him to make you both some warming rum coffees before you rug up together around the warmth.

With no disturbances or interruptions other than the snapping and crackling of the fire, sit entwined, without the pressure of sex, and simply enjoy the time together alone. Sitting alone together, with no interruptions, for an unscheduled amount of time is rare in couples' lives, so drink it in. Let your familiar, warm togetherness seep into every pore.

After you've finished your rum coffees, tell him you've got dessert for him. Either head into the tent or over to your swag and sneak the whipped cream from your bag. Smear it across your breasts with a little "happy trail" leading down your belly to the top of your G-string. Invite him to have a taste of some real bush tucker. Once he's licked you almost clean, kiss his mouth and share in the creamy, sugary sweetness. Undress him and take control like a confident cowgirl. Spread whipped cream on his dick and suck it off; straddle your cowboy and work him in the "ride him cowgirl," woman-on-top position, rocking and swerving your hips as if you were riding a bucking bronco. If you're in a really private area, with no one around for miles, be loud. Whoop it up, shout, scream and moan while no one is around to hear it! When you're both spent, hunker down for the night, naked and wrapped up together in a sleeping bag, and promise him that later in the night, or perhaps at sunrise, you'll tuck in for another bush fuck.

Extra Zing

Take your partner on a blow-job bushwalk—blow his mind by blowing him under a tree. In the dark, lead him to a private tree, making sure no one else is around, and then place a folded blanket by his feet. In the complete darkness, push him against the tree trunk, kiss him, tell him to "*sshhh*," then reach down and unzip his pants. Kneel on the blanket and tell him you're his "lady of the night," in the forest, here to service him in a most primal way. Don't let him touch you—tell him to look at the stars, listen to the bush, and feel enveloped by silence and darkness while he's sucked by your hot, warm, inviting mouth. Occasionally cover your lip-smacking sounds with moans, sighs and hums. As he's about to orgasm, take him deep into your mouth so he comes straight down your throat and past your taste buds. Kiss his shaft, his balls, his pubic hair area and the happy trail up to his navel. Tuck him back into his pants, zip him up, take his hand, give it a kiss, and then lead him back to camp.

Happy trails ... very happy trails!

The Deep South

Explore your southern frontiers.

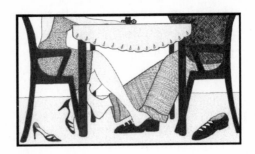

Pleasure Pantry Ingredients
Blindfold (optional)
Massage oil
Feather
Flavored oral sex drops
Pedi spa (optional)
Nail polish (optional)

Preparation
Most of the time when we indulge in a sensual, sexual experience, we explore, touch and caress each other's whole bodies. Foreplay often involves setting alight most main body areas and erogenous zones with desire and titillating, exciting sensation. However, when you restrict touch on particular body areas it can actually heighten the pleasure, as the longer you go without touch on an area, the more you crave to be touched right there. This is the power of our sexual brain, and it's a state that can be maximized in sexual play as you stimulate an area of the body by deliberately ignoring it and making it "out of bounds." The lure of the forbidden leaves you wanting even more.

Create a heightened sensual experience by restricting touch to only one half of the body—the lower half. This means that sexual play is limited to below the waist on each other. No kissing, no arms wrapped around each other, no sensual touch on breasts, necks, chests, hair or faces. All touch must be constrained to the lower half of each other's bodies.

While you might find this boundary constricting at first, soon enough your upper bodies will be simply straining for touch of any kind. It's a sure-fire method to awaken the whole body with desire, while still pleasuring each other's central sexual areas. So get down together and play below the belt ...

Bring to Boil

Begin your natural exploration of each other by getting nude from at least the waist down, although if you're entirely naked from tip to toe it will likely increase the desire to be touched above the navel, and intensify your sexual anticipation in a frustratingly delicious way.

You may wish to boost your partner's awareness of your touch by restricting their senses even further with a blindfold. This way their expectation of where you might go next further eroticizes your touch when and where you do touch them.

Stimulate your lovee's mind by first getting to their sole ... give each other foot reflexology. It may help to get a book on foot reflexology so you can look at a diagram as you massage your partner's feet; but if you don't have one, follow these easy instructions ...

With a small amount of massage oil, rub their entire

foot and ankle to lubricate the area. If your partner is particularly ticklish, firm presses are less likely to induce a
ticklish response than light ones. For the reflexology treatment start with their toes. The toes on both the left and
right feet are linked to the head and brain, so by starting
with toe stimulation you ignite the areas directly linked to
the mind.

Move to their heels and press firmly with one or two fingers into each heel pad. The heels connect to the lower back,
and this can help to further relax your lovee, especially if
they are tense with stress (or sexual frustration). From here
you can move slowly to the middle of the feet, where there
are specific areas which mirror the various regions of their
upper body. You may like to tell them which areas of their
body you are stimulating with your seductive, symbolic
massage—this can further heighten their raging desire to be
actually touched on those places, but no, no—not allowed—
not directly, not yet.

Continue touching beneath the little toes on the ball of
the foot, which represent the shoulders, and move towards
the center of the ball of the foot, which reflects the chest
area. The lower end of the ball of the left foot, in the middle,
specifically reaches the heart. The outer edges of the middle
feet connect to the waistline, and the inner arch on the edge
can soothe the spine.

When you reach the lower end of the inner arch, which
represents the genital area, tease them with touch here and
then tease them verbally also. Ask them how ready they are
to be touched on their dick or pussy. Ask them to describe
how intense their desire is to be touched directly there by
you, since you're stimulating those reflexology zones on

them. Once you feel you've taunted them enough, you can then start to move your touch up their legs towards their very real, very wanting, waiting, love zones.

Once their mind is overwhelmed by anticipation and desire, lie next to them or straddle their upper thighs. Take a feather and lightly stroke them up from their ankles into the crease of their groin. The contrast of the light feather touch with the firm foot massage they've just received will spark them into an alert arousal—not to mention the fact that you're now focusing on their more central, direct sexual nerve areas.

Before you satisfy them with the touch they crave on their twitching dick, hard with desire, or vagina wet with want, turn them over and with the feather, stroke the backs of their legs up to their butt; then, using your hands and elbows, give them a deep bottom massage, working from the base of their spine right down into the fleshy part of their lower butt. The buttocks are one of the body's largest muscle areas, so massaging them not only relaxes them but brings blood flow into the entire region.

Invite them to move onto their back once more, and as they turn over take the oral sex drops and lightly squeeze a few onto their dick or pussy. The drops can be any flavor you wish, from berry to vanilla to coconut—you may like to share the same flavor or choose different ones for each other. Then give them the ultimate down-under kiss by licking and tasting every crevice of their southern parts, covering them in flavored oral drops and sucking them off.

When you've pleasured each other in turns, use your hands to bring each other to mutual pleasure at the same time, and then engage in southern comfort by finally penetrating, still concentrating only on down-under touch. Start with her on top, facing away from him. She can reach down and cup his balls, and stroke and press into his perineum (the area of skin behind his balls) as she rides him up and down. When both want to increase the pace, she can lean forward onto her hands and knees, and he can squat or kneel behind her and thrust from behind in cheeky (doggy) style. As he's able to come fast in this position because of his total control and deep thrusting, she can reach down to stimulate her own clitoris to climax using the lingering oral drop liquid as lube.

When you've both peaked with pleasure, share the rest of your downtime together in a full-body embrace, until sleep comes.

Extra Zing

Prolong your sensual play by engaging in some extra-attentive loving: give each other pedicures before you get sexual with each other. You might do this in the afternoon, long before sexually playing, or you might start with pedicures before moving on to foot reflexology and then slowly increasing sexual play. If he doesn't like the idea of a pedicure, tell him it's a "sports pedicure" and that good care of his feet is as important as good care of his face and the rest of his body. (There's no need to paint his toenails unless he wants to be pampered for fun in this way!)

Take turns to wrap each other's feet in hot, damp towels. Exfoliate your partner's feet with a tingling foot scrub and rinse in a pedi spa or tub of warm water. Massage their feet with oil, working all of the oil in; when it's her turn to be pampered, paint her toenails. He can choose the color he most likes to see her in—men rate well-taken-care-of feet, including polished toes, as an important quality in a sexy woman, so encourage him to paint your toes (let him take his time to lavish attention on you and paint carefully) in a color he finds the sexiest to look at. After all, he'll be spending a lot of time looking at them as he pleasures all your sexy southern fronts.

Play Time

Toys 'R' Her

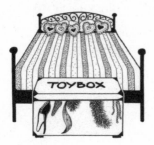

Pleasure Pantry Ingredients

Toys, toys, and more toys! Surf the web, or search your local sex boutique for an array of toys to delight her every sense. A sample toy kit
might include:

   X-rated trivia game
   Soft silicone vibrator
   Smooth egg or bullet vibe with at least seven functions and speeds
   Flavored lube
   Lip gloss tin (stimulating lip gloss for the lower lips)
   Sound-activated vibe
   Rabbit vibe, or vibe/dildo combination—bits that buzz outside as
      well as inside her
   Strap-on clitoris vibe for her to wear
   Penis ring with vibrating clit stimulator
   Miniature tongue vibe
   Scarf

Present of pretty-in-pink lingerie, fluffy heels and fluffy cuffs (optional)
Soft silicone pink vibe (optional)

Preparation

There's a bit of a clichéd joke (which isn't actually that funny),
mainly among women, but also men, that taunts men about

being threatened by the "almighty dildo." The well-used line is that toy play is just for women because men "can't handle the truth": that when it comes to sex, and especially orgasm, women prefer their playthings to their partners when it comes to bedroom play time.

Not true.

In fact, *so* not true that the sex toy industry is booming with couple toys, for both his and her pleasure *together*. The myth that sex toys are for women only, and that men fear and loathe vibrators is simply that: an old—very old—myth.

Modern times have brought about modern sexplay. There are now sound-activated toys; flash toys that plug into your USB port on your computer; toys with more than twenty different functions and speeds; toys that buzz silently yet intensely; vibes for her to wear against her body for "hands-free" pleasure; vibes for him to wear; toys with matching attachments for both to wear, with corresponding remotes for each to operate on the other—and more. It's an exhaustive assortment!

Interestingly, though, despite the plethora of sex accessories in the world today, some stubborn connotations about sex toys as "sex aids"—helpful only when a sex life has gone stale—are still alive and well. But this has not been the case. In fact, the term "dildo" is believed to have derived from the Italian *diletto*, meaning "to delight." Sex accessorizing has, from its origins, been about delight, pleasure and play—not functional assistance (though it can be helpful in that regard, too).

Let this adult recreation session together be all about her: make her your plaything, and tease and delight her. Make her your vibrating Venus of lurve. Use your selection of toys to play with her all over her body. Show her that you not only aren't threatened by toys, vibes and dildos, but that you're willing to give her ultimate pleasure with a wide variety of them under your own direction.

Prepare for your night by getting all your toys in order so you can surprise her with a night of slow-burning, smoldering, buzzing sex unlike any other. Game on! Play! Because as the sex docs say: "Partners who play together, stay together."

Bring to Boil

With your toys bought and stashed (batteries tested and ready) in a bag or adult-version toy box under the bed, invite your lovee to a night to remember. Tell her that you've bought her something but that she has to guess what it is. Reach for a scarf (or soft eye mask) as a blindfold and ask her to close her eyes. Reach down and pull out the X-rated trivia game. Pull off her blindfold and show it to her. At this point she's likely to be extremely disappointed, but she may or may not show it. She was probably thinking that all the suspense would lead to something romantic or super-sexy, not a little trivia game.

If she's quizzical, explain that you're going to play a little game tonight. For every answer she gets right, she gets another sexy surprise. And to keep the entire evening a surprise, she's going to be blindfolded the entire time. She must concentrate on your voice to listen to the questions if she wants to keep experiencing the sexy surprises.

Blindfold her again and lay your toys out within easy reach. Start your game by asking her questions from the X-rated trivia game. (If you didn't, or couldn't, buy the game at your local sex boutique or online, you can prepare some sexy questions about your love life, each other's sexual preferences and your erotic sexual history together. Write them on decorated cards, spread around the bed among the toys, to delightfully surprise her when you take off her blindfold. Include questions like "Where was the first place we ever made love?" "How many countries have we had sex in?" and "What is my favorite color on you?") Each time she answers a question correctly, reach for a toy and buzz it against her skin. Be sure to use a wide variety of toys, and to start with, use them only on her upper body's erogenous zones. As she becomes aroused, travel further south and begin teasing her against her clitoris, through clothes. If she's not wearing any, make sure you apply some lube before pressing a vibe against her, as vibrators can cause friction that can be painful if she's not very wet.

As she gets increasingly excited, start alternating your play between toys, and your fingers and mouth. Keep your variety unpredictable so she never knows what's coming next. You might intensify your play by leaving several vibes on her body at once: strap on a clitoral vibe, press one against her nipple, tuck one under her lower back, and every once in a while activate them at differing speeds all at once, while you kiss and tongue-bathe her.

Challenge yourself to see how many times you can get her to orgasm, in how many different ways. Then let your dick bring her to climax without entering her but, rather, rubbing head to head, dick to clit, with both of you sharing the buzzing vibrator sensations. And when she is quivering with pleasure-pulses of orgasm, plunge into her wet vag and get yourself off too, while she's still throbbing with satisfaction. When it's all over, pull off her blindfold and reveal to her, at last, all the pleasure tools that made your sex such a pleasurable playtime. And on and on.

Extra Zing

Take her to another level of pleasure by really grasping total control of the night and theme.

Think pink, all the way. Give her a present in a beautifully wrapped long box tied with a big pink bow, and six or twelve pink roses attached. Inside the box, meticulously wrapped in tissue paper, she'll find a gorgeous negligee set, in pink, with coordinating satin panties and matching slip-on kitten heels, complete with fluffy open toes (these are available from online female-friendly passion-party toy shops). Her new outfit carries with it the essence of glamor-puss from tip to toe, so ask her to swan around in it for you and show herself off.

Give her the opportunity to feel indulged and special with your thoughtfulness before you present her with the last item of her gift. Take her to the bed, lay her down and begin kissing her. As she's being swept away with your romance, reach for the fluffy pink plush cuffs and snap one onto her wrist with a smile. Tease her with the other one, and when she's in a comfortable position (this is about indulgence, pampering and flirtatious control, not strict S & M), tie up her other wrist. Your porn-Barbie sweetie is now good enough to eat, dressed prettily in fluff and pink, ready to be ravished. Take a brand-new vibe (a soft silicone, baby-doll pink one if you can find it) and tickle her from her inner arms to her breasts, through her negligee, down to her navel, across and around her inner thighs, and then through her satin panties. Reach for a tin of sexual "lip gloss" and put a little on your fingers before reaching into her panties. Apply this lower-lip gloss to lube her up for play, and then move the vibe into her panties. Enjoy the sight of your gorgeous glamorpuss dressed in sexy diva retro fluff and satin, writhing under your power-enhanced touch. Take your time to pleasure her—she's all tied up. Your damsel in delight.

The Rain Check

Ultimate make-up sex

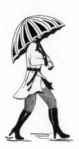

Pleasure Pantry Ingredients
Full-length raincoat
His favorite lingerie to see on her
High-heeled shoes
Pen and paper

Preparation
While well over half of all women and men would prefer more sex, the fact of the matter is that life can get in the way of an ideal, frequent-encounter sex life. Sometimes people are too tired, stressed or busy to engage in sex ... or they really *do* have a headache!

While both men and women turn down sex, for one reason or another, international research and anecdotal evidence reveals that women do so more often (but this may simply be because men are more noisy complainers about this than women, and so may not accurately reflect the truth).

Sex is a vital part of a passionate relationship, and connecting through physical intimacy can become a barometer of how happy and satisfied a couple's union is. However, research shows that it's not how often a couple has sex that is the most important ingredient, but how valued, appreciated, adored and desired each partner feels that is more crucial. And this is where make-up sex fits in.

It's a simple fact that, at some point in a relationship, one partner is going to want sex when the other doesn't or simply isn't in the mood. This is perfectly natural. How the couple deals with this sexual incompatibility, and how they make up for it, becomes the more important gauge of the health of their overall relationship.

Make-up sex after a fight is often intense, passionate and needy, as partners desire to reconnect and reaffirm their bond after conflict. What becomes a little more difficult to navigate is finding your way back to passion after one partner has rejected an initiation (or many) for sex, without conflict, and even without explanation.

Taking a "rain check" for sex means making up for sex that has previously been rejected. Like taking a rain check for anything else, it means that you're willing to reschedule the experience for a later time. When it comes to sex, though, because rejection can be sorely felt, a rain check means make-up sex times ten, injecting your lovemaking with hot passion to satiate the "rejected" partner's every desire. You don't want to just make up for the sex session that was missed, but reassure your partner that you do desire them as much as you ever have, by making it sex they'll never forget. So when you want to pull out all the stops, Rain Check sex means engaging in all your partner's favorite things . . .

For the purposes of this Rain Check, it's her making it up to him. But if he's been the one to take a rain check . . . come up with your own saucy variation! To prepare, make sure you have a full-length raincoat, lingerie that you know he loves to see you in, and prepare a written list of the top ten reasons why you love and desire him.

Bring to Boil

You know your partner best, and you know which sexual buttons to push. You can decide whether you want to surprise your partner with a Rain Check, or whether you entice him with flirty messages and hints that "tonight is the night." Regardless, embody the Rain Check theme by wearing lingerie that you know is his favorite to see on you, with simply a raincoat over the top and nothing but high heels showing at the bottom. Make him curious about what you've got on underneath—a full outfit, or nothing at all?

Meet him at his office, a hotel, or at the front door, and give him a teasing flash of you in his favorite lingerie and nothing else under the coat. Kiss him and let him know that you're making good on your rain check for previously not responding to sex when he wanted it. A man's ego likes to be stroked as much as his body, especially if it's been a bit quashed through previous sexual rejection, so show your true sexual desire for him by first expressing it through words, and not just action.

Tell him to sit down and then, as you stand before him, coat draped open to reveal a hint of what's underneath, reach into the pocket of your coat and pull out your list of what you love and desire about him. Read your list very slowly, and make sure that it builds to a sexual crescendo. If your list includes things like "I love you because you're a good father, you take care of our family, you're a wonderful provider," then escalate to the sexual side of your relationship, expressing your love for him in ways like "You make me feel beautiful, your body is hot, especially when I get to see it in the morning when you're showering and the water spills over you. I love your arms around me, your smile makes me melt, and when you tease me in bed, I can't help but want more. Your dick is the only thing that can utterly satisfy me. I miss your smell when you aren't with me . . ." Use your own words to express your thoughts, but keep them specific to your partner—make it all about him. He'll be craving and loving the attention you're giving him while standing nearly nude, literally exposing yourself to him, and knowing without a doubt that you want, desire, love and adore him.

After you've read your top ten reasons for being hot for him, tell him that this make-up sex session is also all about him. Everything and anything he wants. You may like to dominate the session, knowing his premier preferences, or you may want to ask him what he'd like, given the spontaneous heat of the moment. Go with it. Make the most of it.

Extra Zing

Talk as a couple about incorporating the concept of Rain Check sex into your love life. Acknowledge that it's natural for your sexual gears to be misaligned from time to time, and that when one partner wants to get their gear off, the other may not. This doesn't always have to be the stereotype of the man constantly wanting sex—women want, and get rejected for, sex from their partner too. Negotiating a pact for rain-check sex allows for flexibility in a couple's sex life, acknowledges that there will be times when either partner isn't in the same mood, and allows for an avenue in which rejection is okay—not personal, but simply a reflection of outward circumstances or uncontrolled moods, lack of sleep, hormones, stress—et cetera! Open communication about the lack of sex in a relationship only serves to heat it up, especially if partners are well aware of "Plan B."

You may like to help your sex life go from drought to drench by creating a Rain Check envelope and placing it in your bedside table drawer. Both of you write down three sexual things you'd like to have done by your partner on separate pieces of paper, and place those six pieces of paper in the envelope. Then, whenever a partner rejects sex, the other can say, "Are you asking for a Rain Check?," knowing that there is an envelope of Rain Check alternatives to draw from at the next available time. Then the next day or week, the rain-check partner draws one out to indulge in. Sample Rain Check coupons include:

Blow job in the shower

Dinner and a night at a hotel

30-minute bath together

Watch a porn movie with me

Have sex on top of me

Buy me a new toy

Go down on me and give me three orgasms

Use a sex toy on me

Give me an erotic massage

Read me an erotic bedtime story

Tie me up and have your way with me

Tease me for an hour until I come.

Desire? Check. Satisfaction? Check.

Sizzling

Shall we play?
Let's not be gentle tonight ...
Let it sting
a little.
You know what they say about
fine lines,
pleasure,
pain ...

Fire and Ice

Cool lovers make a hot combination.

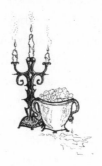

Pleasure Pantry Ingredients
Blindfold or eye pillow
Blanket
Heating pads
Heating oil (purchased in most sex shops)
Ice cubes
Peppermint tea
Flavored ice blocks
Lit candle on a bedside table
Vibrator
Lube
Sauna (optional)

Preparation
Prepare for a total skin-centric emphasis on heightening arousal through unpredictable touch and contrasting sensations. Setting the skin alight inflames the mind—and your desire for more of your lover's touch—even more, and inspires even deeper touch, on and in each other. Flicker each other into a frenzied sexual state of need for each other with shivering cold strokes and burning hot blows. The only

preparation needed is to have your ingredients at hand, so you have immediate access to the contrasting stimulators.

Bring to Boil

Remembering that unpredictable touch is the key, blindfold the receiver. This way the emphasis is on their sense of touch, as they can't see which ingredients you're reaching for to use on them next. But if your partner isn't comfortable being totally restricted in this way, use an eye pillow instead.

Start by warming them to get their blood flowing—you don't want to begin with cooling touch because the objective is to get them hot and sexually stimulated, which requires increased blood flow. Lay your lovee down, facing up, and place a blanket over them; tell them to relax. Quickly microwave a couple of heating pads and then place them under your lovee's neck and the small of their back—this will immediately start the warming and relaxation of their body.

Take the heating oil and rub it up and down their chest, shoulders, arms, belly, waist, navel, across their hips, and down their legs and thighs. Once in a while, lean over and blow on particular areas, especially unexpected ones such as their inner forearms, ribcage, hip bones and inner thighs. The heating oil will increase in temperature as soon as you blow on it. Tease them by rubbing this same oil over their genitals, but avoid blowing on their lower sexy areas at this point—give them a hint of the sensation that may come, but don't satisfy them with it yet.

When they're feeling red hot, alternate touch by reaching for an ice cube and trickle it down their throat, towards and over their nipples, and down, in and around their navel. Slide the melting ice cube down their hips and thighs; run it back up their inner thighs and lightly across their groin.

Lean down and lick them with your warm, flat tongue. Then take a sip of hot peppermint tea from the cup on your bedside table and lick and suck where you just were, with your now even hotter mouth. Some people who are acutely attuned to every sensation and nuance may notice the contrast of the heat with the tingle of the peppermint, while others will have enough blood flowing southwards that all they notice is the searing heat of your lips and mouth.

Kiss your partner's nipples and continue to rub them, and then reach for a flavored ice block (which may be wrapped to keep it frozen during all this prolonged loveplay). Slide it down their torso and across their most sensitive glans, down through their groin to the inner thighs. As it melts, the sugar of the ice block will leave a colored sticky trail ... for you to retrace and lick clean.

Once they're satiated with oral touch, contrast that loving approach with some wicked wax play. With your lovee still lying on their back, turn their head away from the bedside table. Take the lit candle and drip the tiniest bit of wax in minute droplets down their back. Hot wax on the skin produces a micro-instant of searing, alert pain, followed by expanding warmth on the skin, and then a tightening feeling as the wax quickly dries. Couples not usually into S & M can find this an exotic, potentially erotic, sudden sensation. Use the wax minimally, for only a few drops. Let it serve as a contrast, not a primary stimulant.

Then immediately gratify your partner sensually with kisses and strokes, and re-lube them again with the heating oil on other areas of their body, to draw their attention away from where you have just been concentrating. Twist them back onto their front and straddle them, now ready to use a vibrator (prepared with lube) to really heat them up. Using a light pressure, give them tingling sensations with the vibe down their arms and on their nipples, and lightly blow everywhere you just touched them with the vibrator to further add a cool shiver. When you reach their groin, avoid their main sex organ and press the vibe firmly into their inner thighs and upwards into the side crease near their outer lips or balls. This way you can draw heat and sensation to their groin without actually touching their most sensitive parts.

Keep them wanting more and, as their body heats up again, rub more heating oil on their glans and surrounding areas, then blow long, cooling breaths and hot, wide, short breaths, to ignite the heating oil on their most sensitive nerve endings.

When you both can't stand any more, lie side by side, facing each other, as he penetrates; holding your bodies close to create warmth and share your sweat and scent. Thrust against each other in tandem, creating maximum in-and-out movement, and then alternate this by swivelling both your hips so you grind against each other. This grinding motion not only creates heat but can provide pubic stimulation which sometimes reaches the erect clitoris. If not, though, use the vibe or one of your hands to bring her to climax before, or as, he peaks. Bask in the glow of your shared heat.

Extra Zing
Increase the intensity by having sex in a sauna. Sweat together, touching each other naked, until you're both slippery wet all

over. Then body-slide up and down your partner, using your genitals as the main instrument of touch. Once you've slid your bodies all over each other, using your sweat—perhaps with added lube or oil—engage in sweaty, slick sex sitting up, with her on his lap, facing him. Both of you use muscles in this position which circulate more blood as you work out, create more physical heat between you, and better enable both of you to come.

Soak in each other's lust, and swivel in a mutual rhythm until you're spent. With your glowing bodies and relaxed muscles replete with pleasure, slide down between the cool, crisp sheets of your bed for a well-deserved deep sleep, filled with warm, wet dreams of your fiery hunger for each other, satiated.

Picture It

Make love to the camera.

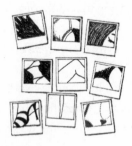

Pleasure Pantry Ingredients
Digital camera (with self-timer)
Men's tie
Lingerie
Video camera/digital movie cam
Cell phone camera (optional)

Preparation
Set a date so both of you can have your bodies primped and primed for the occasion. Think "erotic art," not "porn," for this session together, and through visual expression, celebrate the beauty of your body union.

Many people can be self-conscious about having their picture taken—especially naked!—however, the idea of this time together is to have fun and record the memory. It's recommended that this be a daytime activity as the dark requires flash photography, and each crack of a flash can snap your lovee back into "oh-I'm-being-photographed" mode, breaking the reverie you share together. A nice afternoon sun often provides a glowing and flattering light, or else the morning can result in some oh-so-sexy, rumpled, carefree, sexy, tousled bed-head shots.

If you're feeling even braver, take shots of each other outside the bedroom. Find a sexy location that means something to the both of you—perhaps go back to the hotel where you shared your honeymoon, or go to a hotel on the same block as where you had your first date, or go outdoors—just so long as you're in your private garden of pleasure: this sensuous recipe isn't designed for the spicy kick of getting arrested!

Bring to Boil

If you or your partner is shy, make the situation more comfortable by photographing them wrapped in sheets, or behind a few pillows or in a robe. Give them a range of loving-to-hot reassurances, telling them how gorgeous they are. You don't have to go as far as posing like models do, or mimic professional photographers oozing "Work it baby, yeah, make love to the camera," unless you want to.

You can also create several moods by being serious and coy with the camera, or silly and giggling—it's entirely up to you, and your idea of the private moments you create and catch.

Use the stills camera first to take shots of your lovee's face and body. Take pictures in black and white, or simply develop some in black and white to later make a private erotic album of the two of you.

Start with non-genital shots of each other, and have a play with artistic expressions of your erotica. Try taking a picture of something like her fist clasping his tie, with her painted nails against his chest with an open shirt and one of her nipples dropped into the background. Or a shot of his mouth kissing her closed eyelids. These aren't designed to be "perfect" photos—don't think you're competing with what a professional photographer would achieve. In fact, the more amateurish, blurry and off-center the better, in a sense, because the images will be an accurate reflection of how you see each other, not someone else's outside perception of you.

When you're comfortable and full with love from the camera celebration of other's skins and souls, move on to photographing each other fully nude during the act of your love. You can snap each other giving hand and oral pleasure or capture your serene, radiant faces, satisfied right after orgasm, with shots taken by one of you or with a self-timer. Have sex in the woman-on-top position, as it can better allow both partners to hold the camera and click, mid-sex, with graphic views of you both.

Taking pictures of each other's faces and pelvic union during sex can capture not only a private moment but illuminate your partner's beauty while they are experiencing their "sex flush." During the sexual response, both men and women experience "sex skin," which is a deepening flush of color on various parts of their body, from face, neck, chest to belly, penis and vulva, even thighs and feet. Capturing this sex flush on film can get your mind racing back to that same arousal every time you look at the picture.

If you choose to take pictures of each other on separate cameras, once you have them developed (easily done at home these days to avoid embarrassing trips to the chemist to pick up the developed sexy photos) each of you can choose a few and then privately write some captions on photo album paper. Then, one evening, sit in bed together and combine your individual photo pages into an album of the two of you, sharing with each other what you wrote about each other beside the pictures. Captions may include phrases like "You're most beautiful in the morning, looking straight at me with that smile" and "I love your arms the most, and even more when they're wrapped around me." Make your captions personal, complimentary and sensuous. With your words, you can add a dimension of memory and feeling to the visual. Your love and desire for each other will be forever imprinted: right there in black and white.

Extra Zing

You can add extra sizzle to your erotic album by taking explicit pictures of each other's hottest erotic bits. You can also add poems, words of lust, drawings and personal mementos to make your erotic album a tribute to the sexy side of your relationship.

If you really want to get a bit rude with your nude shots of each other, take a few of you using your partner's mobile phone and leave them on there as a surprise. The phone-cam shots can serve as a personal, very at-hand, erotic remembrance of you—however, this sizzle comes with some caution. If you surprise your partner, tell them straightaway to check their phone to see what you left for them—don't run the risk of them opening their phone in company, especially inappropriate company! Also, don't leave explicit shots on the phone if you're at all worried about security, trust, or others' (i.e. kids/coworkers) access to it. Rather, take a more obscure picture of one of your body parts. Even the most subtle nude shot can have your lovee snapping to your attention!

Center Stage

The strip-and-tease show for him.

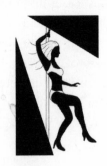

Pleasure Pantry Ingredients

Video/DVD: *Showgirls, Strip Tease*
Costumes—lingerie, top, outfit
Music
Pole-dancing lessons (optional)
Pole (optional)
Video—for rehearsal (optional)

Preparation

Perform a striptease for your partner to give him the show of his life. If you've never stripped, or danced, for your partner (as opposed to with your partner) before, this can be a daunting idea. Get naked slowly and slinkily, to music, without laughing? It can give the strongest of women anxious heart palpitations. But you can do it! It's all about confidence.

Don't worry about intricate, sexy choreographed rhythms and your body shape—those are secondary considerations way, way down the list. You'll be a success at stripping if you can channel all your powers of seductive confidence while you do it. And if you don't feel confident, here's the big secret: this is one situation where it's okay to fake. After all, many strippers fake something every night! As soon as you start pretending you're confident, you'll get into the role and you'll then gain *real* confidence. Your confidence will also soar when you see your lover watching you with wide eyes and an eager grin.

Confidence won't simply magically appear, though, so having the right outfit to strip out of is a critical part of the show. After all, he's watching you ... but he's also paying attention to the pieces of clothing you remove, one by one. So to prepare for this striptease, find an outfit that will make you feel sexy and help you tap into a persona that has confidence. If you feel shy, channel your inner vamp. If you feel you don't have an inner vamp, watch some stripping videos to help create some ideas—you could watch *Strip Tease* starring Demi Moore, or *Showgirls* for ideas.

There's no rule that says you have to strip all the way to fully nude—this is your show, so you get to decide where it begins and where it ends. If you're not happy about showing your belly area, think about stripping down to a halfway unbuttoned shirt of his, with a sexy choker necklace and thigh-high hosiery which you then roll down, slowly. If you're not happy with your bottom, consider stripping out of a dress to reveal a sheer sexy slip with a higher-than-thigh-high slit and peekaboo panties, thigh-high boots and a beautiful bra. Your costuming is key: it's a visual feast for your partner, so it's important to pay attention to what you're wearing—for his eyes, and to enhance your best features.

Bring to Boil

Once you've chosen your costume, it's time to dance. There are few strict rules in a good striptease; the dancing is about open interpretation, but it's worth bearing in mind the famous words of legendary stripper, dancer and performer Gypsy Rose Lee: "Anything worth doing is worth doing slowly." Your heart might be racing, revving you up to 'take it all off' rather quickly, but make sure you slow yourself down. Pick music that you feel sexy moving to, and spend some time just dancing to it (whether you're practicing or performing) without trying to remove any clothing—get into the sexy soul of the song.

Before the event, pick a few moves, only a few, and choreograph them to the slower and faster parts of the song. Don't try to get complicated—the more natural it feels to you, the sexier it will be for him. Remember: you only need about five moves throughout the whole song. He's not going to notice because, as far as he's concerned, the show changes with every article you remove! Moves can include sexy, slow shoulder rotations and hip swivels. The hip swivel has many variations such as these top ten (but there are even more): 1) legs together; 2) legs apart; 3) one leg in front of the other in a modelesque pose; 4) butt pouting out back; 5) hips shifting side to side like a hula girl; 6) grinding and swinging front and back; 7) looping your hips around in a full-circle Hula Hoop style; 8) swivelling a figure-eight pattern; 9) dropping your knees down low and wriggling your hips back up to standing height; 10) slow side swoops and fast twitches like a belly dancer.

And of course don't forget to include your desirous, sultry facial expressions—you can communicate a lot with your eyes and face. Slowly put your fingers in your mouth, through your hair and around your clothes. Don't let him touch you—only *you* get to do the touching.

Give him some peeks at you by quickly spreading your legs in front of him, but don't—repeat, *do not*—let him touch, and don't let him see too much. This is a strip*tease*, before it's a strip-*take me*.

Once you've danced to the song, spend the first part of the second song undressing him. Make him scorch with sticky-hot desire for you. Then finish as you started: with you in control, on top of center stage.

Extra Zing

To really get your lover sizzling under his collar, pole dance for him. Pole dancing is gaining popularity, so join in: get lessons, secretly, and then surprise him with a show. Most pole-dancing studios will have you confident with a routine within a few weeks, and you'll get incredibly fit in the process. Many studios also sell retractable poles which you can buy and fit in your own home.

Let your pole-dancing instructor know that you're planning to surprise your partner with a show, and they'll help you develop a routine. Make sure you've picked a song with the right tempo to allow for the moves suited to your level of pole skill. Once you've got your routine memorized, practice, practice, practice. Pole dancing takes huge skill and strength, and to truly impress your man you want to be confident with every amazing move. Spend a few minutes each day visualizing yourself on the pole, picturing your moves, and tapping into your skilfully sexy dancer persona.

Thinking along the lines of positive visualization not only increases your confidence, but develops a shortcut in your mind to arouse that dirty dancin' girl to the front and center of your brain. This will ignite further when you're actually in costume and start your dance for him.

You may choose to get a retractable pole, and, if you do, set it up (or have a friend help) in the lounge or bedroom while your lovee is out at work. Practice a few times on your new pole and make sure you're dressed in your hot outfit when he comes home. Listen for when he arrives, and as he comes through the door start some warm-up moves on the pole, pretending that he's catching you unawares. When he's "sprung" you, sit your big boy down for a treat.

If setting up your own pole in your home is too impractical, speak to your pole-dancing instructor about variations to use in your home. If dancing for your partner under the light of the moon in your back yard, on your clothesline or swing set, loses some of its appeal, you can look to give your lover a lunchtime breather (heavy breather!) by inviting him to meet you for lunch, and instead lead him to a strip club. You can pay to rent a studio or private booth, where you can then tease him with your solo show. If you can't find a strip club that will rent out space, or you're self-conscious about dancing in a public strip club (mid-afternoon can be a slow time, but rarely are the clubs ever empty), ask your instructor if they rent out their studios when not giving lessons. Once you've found the right "where" and "when"—and you certainly know "how"—pole dance your way into his pants.

Porn Utopia

XXX sex—starring you

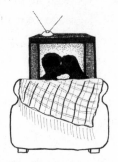

Pleasure Pantry Ingredients
Porn videos/DVDs (a selection for her and for him)
Erotica CD of hot bedtime stories
Cock ring
Sex toy (a couple vibrator for him and her together recommend)
Lube
Video camera and tape

Preparation
Playing with porn as a couple can sometimes be confronting for both men and women. Men might find it unusual and perhaps uncomfortable to share the experience of watching porn with a female partner, since for many men it is a solo indulgence. Women might find porn objectionable or under-whelming in the arousal stakes; or, more commonly, find that women in porn films are competition to live up to with their partner. They can worry that their partner is comparing them to the girls on film, or that he will expect them to behave like a porn star, and that can create some serious per-formance pressure. Rather than viewing porn as a serious

encounter, simply have some fun playing together, with the porn films as a vehicle for shared sexplay.

If porn is seen as a primary source of sex education—especially some sort of education in "how to pleasure a woman"—it often falls far short of reality. A lot of women do not pant, groan or moan anything like the women in porn do. Porn films are notoriously shot as a male fantasy, focus chiefly on his pleasure, concentrate on the "in and out," and rarely show the length and variety of how to realistically satiate a woman sexually.

When indulging in porn together, see it for what it is: a visual turn-on and an accessory to your lovemaking. Both women and men have hard-wiring in their brains to appreciate visual sexual stimuli, although men tend to appreciate and respond to it a bit more—but it's a myth that women can't be turned on by porn. If you prepare for this playtime together with a variety of porn films—some that she may like, and others for his tastes alone—it's more likely you'll both get hot watching and wanking together.

Bring to Boil

Tease out the evening by delaying your foray into film for a bit. Start your raunchy fun by having a bath together or giving each other massages as you listen to an erotic CD of sexy bedtime stories. This auditory stimulation will prime your anticipation for sex, and for watching it. Once you're wet, and hot, settle yourselves in front of the television for some porno indulgence.

As the film gets under way, make touching each other forbidden at the start. As he begins to get hard (it won't usually take long!), he can slip a cock ring on to the base of his shaft to prolong his erection, and you can both extend your play into a second film (or at least the end of the first flick!).

As you watch and touch yourselves, don't get separately engrossed in the film, but rather talk to each other about the effect the film is having on each of you. You may be naked, to see each other fully, or partially dressed with undies around knees or ankles and shoes and tops on. He can tell her how hard he's getting, and she can tell him how wet she feels. Tell the other when something is particularly exciting. If your partner isn't talking, ask them, "Does that make you hot?" Lean over them to get their attention on you and ask, "Do you like what you see?"

When you are *really* horny, but not yet about to come, reach over and stimulate each other as he feels her wetness, and she feels his rock-hard cock. Engage in mutual hand-teases, and then take turns with oral stimulation. She can lick him up and down his shaft, reach one hand up and direct his gaze from the screen down to her holding his cock in her mouth. Then she can lie back and direct his face down so he can suck her clitoris as she watches the film, and also his mouth on her.

Take the couple vibrator toy and place one vibe on each of you. Give each other your corresponding remote, so you can each control the stimulation on the other. While you might both be very wet with her natural lube and his pre-cum, it's always best to add lube whenever playing with a vibe because its motor motion creates so much friction. The lube adds extra slipperiness, and so more stimulation for you both.

Stop and start on each other to create a tactile crescendo while the porn stars are cumming all over each other. Come or not, either or both, but use the couple vibe to play and heighten the eagerness of getting to that ultimate porn-starring climax yourselves. Once you're wild to penetrate, and be penetrated, have him definitely bring her to orgasm—if she hasn't come already—before gaining entry. Her orgasm before penetration will have her at the top of her arousal so that her enjoyment of penetration is maximized, and she might even come again while he's inside her.

Lie down together in the spooning position, both facing the screen, so you can both watch the other stars having sex, orgy-style, as you do it. To amp up your frenzied lovemaking, pull out and switch to the wheelbarrow position, which is rear entry but, instead of having her on her knees, he lifts her legs up as one would the handles of a wheelbarrow. After a few thrusts of this position, switch to the man-on-top position where you can both look down and get a view of your joining together. Immediately the focus of attention will shift from watching others having sex on screen to your personal pornographic experience. It's much hotter to watch each other in the here and now than any porn film, no matter how famous the stars. You have become the stars.

Extra Zing

Make an amateur porn film together, starring both of you. Keep it real—do not act out a fantasy of you both "being porn stars" unless you're both 100 percent comfortable with this. If she's at all anxious or worried about being compared to other porn stars, this could set up a potentially destructive competition which will likely short-circuit her arousal, and she might end up resenting the whole experience. Stay on the side of safe porn sex by making a film of you two as yourselves.

Before you enter the world of amateur porn, discuss the practicalities first. This isn't sexy, but it's vital to being able to really let go during the filming experience together, once you've decided what will happen to the tape. If you agree to keep the "evidence" private, to be shared only ever between the two of you, make sure you also agree on a secret hiding place for the tape. Label the tape something innocuous but meaningful to you both, and ensure that you both agree to its storage—or that you both agree to erase it after a set amount of time (a week, a month, three months—longer than this and you run the risk of it being potentially discovered by someone, plus if you erase it after three months it gives you a sexy incentive to make another!).

You could add even more sizzle by venturing into cyberporn. You can create a website dedicated to your sex together, including photos, videos and saucy passages of eroticism to each other—even making up porn names for each other which you use anytime you're on the site, separately or apart … your porno alter egos! This is only practical if the site is absolutely and completely locked with an access code that only you two know (unless you want to share your porn alter egos publicly!).

Research the security angles thoroughly before even contemplating this idea and negotiate a trust agreement before uploading anything. The upshot: you can see each other having sex any time you go online, from anywhere in the world, which can be incredibly steamy if you're ever apart. The downside: your personal money shots could be seen by others if the security isn't tight enough. If you do go cyberpornographic together, explore the new frontier to its full fucking potential.

Ecstasy and Agony

Hanky spanky: the union of pleasure and pain.

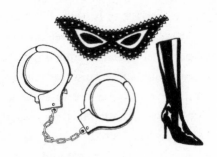

Pleasure Pantry Ingredients
Handcuffs (with snap-lock release)
Stiletto boots
Ping pong bat or sex paddle
Leather sex whip or belt
Leather collar
Feathers
Soft mitt
Scratchy mitt
Black lingerie
Clothes pegs
Cock ring
Black leather bra with nipple cutouts (optional)
Scissors (optional)

Preparation
Exploring the world of bondage and domination (B & D) shouldn't be entered into completely spontaneously the first time, especially if you've never talked together as a couple about whether either of you like the idea. If you're completely new to the world of BDSM (bondage, discipline and

sadomasochism), take a trip together to a sex shop that has a variety of specially designed toys for fetish sex. You don't necessarily have to buy anything—you can simply get some ideas for the kind of play you might like to experiment with. It's relatively easy to introduce each other to the world of B & D with budget items and household goods before you venture out to purchase specially made B & D accessories. For example, you can use a spatula or ping pong bat instead of a sex paddle; a small, light, buckle-free leather belt instead of a sex whip or clothes pegs instead of nipple clamps.

To *really* spark your imagination for the wide, weird and wonderful range of possible stimulations, a visit to a sex shop might be helpful. As you look over the range together, tell each other then—and afterwards in late-night whispers—the things that appeal and those that don't. This will give you an even better idea of the boundaries that you can play within, with each other. This is also a good point at which to discuss your safe words. All bondage and domination play must involve consent at every stage. To ensure this, agree on using the word "yellow" for "Caution, I'm nearing my limit" and "red" for "Stop now." Don't use words like "stop," "don't" or "no," because these words can be uttered in sexual ecstasy and might be misinterpreted. "Yellow" and "red" are clear and easy to remember, and aren't generally run-of-the-mill sexual reflex words.

Once you've agreed to try B & D, you need to decide which roles you're going to play. Men often prefer to be dominated, because they're used to being in control and often take the initiative in sex. Some clients of professional Mistresses are successful, controlling businessmen who find that "letting go" and submitting to a dominating partner liberates their mind and body, and that creates a more acute sense of pleasure, precisely because they are out of control and not able to determine what comes next. So, while you can switch roles in your B & D play, start the first evening with giving her all the power.

She can dictate the time and the place, and she can do so in advance to drive him crazy with curious and exciting anticipation. Pack a pair of handcuffs in his briefcase before he goes to work, and attach a note: "You're going to be wearing these by 9 p.m. Prepare to submit to my every desire."

If it's not practical to include cuffs in his work bag, you can lay out all the items you intend on wearing and using on the bed, take a digital photo of them and email or mms it to him with a similar note—or simply no text, but with the subject heading "Tonight."

Bring to Boil

When he comes home, be wearing your Fuck Me stiletto boots and a sexy black outfit of your choice—black is the color of domination, so embrace it; be the Mistress of the house. You are in control from the word go and the creak of the front door. Don't let routines like dinner and the evening news stop you—have your session now. Be assertive. (You can enjoy a meal once you're otherwise satiated, and relax over the late-night news.)

Approach him and demand the handcuffs from his briefcase (or have them in your grasp if you didn't send him off with them in the morning). Order him to sit down and place his hands in his lap. Cuff him, then sit on his lap and move his cuffed hands to your pussy and demand that he rub you through your clothes. Bark at him to stop when you want him to.

Get off him, and circle around him. You may want a prop like a paddle, whip or belt to play with in your hands as you speak to him. Tell him he's been very bad, and that he's going to be punished until you're satisfied. Be serious: you are the disciplinarian. If you feel you're about to break character (because the role can feel new to you), lean down and tell him to reach up and kiss you. Order him to touch and kiss any part of you that you like. But don't pleasure him yet—starting with the emphasis on you makes him wait, and waiting pushes him even further into submission.

When you're ready to start a tactile tease on him, take a pair of scissors and cut the front of his shirt so you can rip it off of him. Rip with abandon. (If you don't want to rip his shirt, take it off him, undo his handcuffs and sternly order him to sit still, on his hands.) Get off on restraining him and controlling his every movement with just your whim and voice.

Put a leather collar around his neck. You may not do anything with it—this time—but wearing it will nail his impression that he is being dominated—you own him.

Scratch his back with your fingers and nails, and then contrast this sensation with a feather lightly tickled down his back and chest. Continue to alternate hard and soft touches with all your toys at hand, especially the soft and scratchy mitts. Instruct him when you want to be touched, then hand him the instrument of play and tell him exactly where and how he's to pleasure you with it.

Order him to stand, and unzip him and take off his trousers. Yank them down roughly, then spank his bottom.

Reach for the paddle and give him a few harder spanks through his underwear. Pull down his underwear and ask him if he'd like you to touch his dick. Make a motion to do so, then tell him he has to wait—you have more in store for him yet. While he watches, strip down to your lingerie; take off your panties and drape them down his face, under his nose and across his mouth, then tie them around his leather collar so that the smell of your sex wafts up to him.

Take a few clothes pegs and snap a few on his ear lobes, then release, to give him the sensation of instant pinching pressure. Before you squeeze the pegs anywhere else, test them on your hand, on the skin between your thumb and fore-finger, to double check that they aren't too pinching—you want to achieve a light squeeze, not true agony. Place them on his fingers, toes, nipples and anywhere else that takes your fancy. Don't leave any one peg on too long, though—this is beginner fetish sex, and you want to gradually build up sensation, not douse him in pain until he turns off.

Order him to tell you how sexy you are. Tell him (don't ask—*demand*) to list all your sexy qualities. Remember, dominating a man should be erotic and rewarding for you, too, not just an exercise in wildly pleasing him.

With both of you standing, take the sex whip and lightly whip him across his butt and back. You don't want to cause anything more than instantaneous pain because lasting pain can shut off the sexual response, and that would be counter-productive to this kind of play.

After all this, stand in front of him and reach down to hold his dick in your hands. As you rub his erection, or bring him to erection if he's soft or semi-hard, put a cock ring on the base of his dick to help him last longer and feel every inch of pleasure as you continue to tease his shaft and balls. Then tell him to get down on his knees and lick you till you come.

Push him down and get on top of him. Ride him until you want to switch gears, then get off him and order him back onto his knees. Bend over in front of him and tell him to fuck you from behind, cheeky doggy style, until he blows. Tell him to spank you as he pushes in you, but he's only to spank you when you say.

Tell him to tidy up the sex mess while you shower. Walk off in your fucking sexy boots, and look back with a smile and tell him he's a good boy.

Extra Zing

To liven up your B & D play even more, live the dominatrix/ submissive personas for an entire day, not just the night. Get into each of your roles by ordering him around, and by him submitting to your every demand.

You can dictate, from the morning on, what he should wear—from his outer wear to his underwear. You can send him email and phone messages to tell him what to expect that night, and to order him to touch himself at specific points in the day. You can tell him exactly when to arrive home, and threaten that you will not be pleased if he's even a minute late.

Live the roles throughout the day so you can embrace the sense of dominating, and he the feeling of being dominated. The roles will feel even more real when you come together to play them out sexually that night, and the torment of antic- ipation all day long will heighten the sensory experience when you are finally together.

To enhance the experience even further, you can book in with a professional Mistress to get tips on how to professionally drive him painfully happy. Many Mistresses don't just take on their regular clients for domination, but also run "Reform Schools" and wicked workshops for women, to train them how to take control of their sex lives and dominate their men at home. Let your fingers do the walking to find one near you, and then when you have really, skilfully learned how, let your hips and lips to do the talking.

Oh, the agony! Oh oh oh—the ecstasy!

Tarzan and Jane

Swing into each other and fulfill your primal urges.

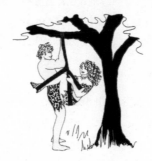

Pleasure Pantry Ingredients
Rotating sex swing (available from sex shops)
Candles
Animal-print lingerie
Music
Vibrator
Blindfold

Preparation

You might not be swinging from vines, or even swinging from a chandelier, but you can have swinging sex, just the two of you, in a rotating love swing. It's best to purchase a specially made sex swing rather than try to construct one yourselves, although a hammock can also be substituted (however more balance may be required so you don't tip over!). A specially made sex swing can give you the option to explore positions that defy gravity, and have you and your partner spinning and sparking with fun-filled fucking.

Sex swings are flexible and sturdy, usually hinge on a steel spring which allows 360-degree rotation, and have helpful features such as rotating stirrups, padded seats and a handlebar for leverage. They can easily hook up and then be dismantled for discreet play.

A sex swing allows for sexperimentation and a true novelty factor; it's not usually a serious staple in a couple's love life, but it can add a bit of a kinky twist for a thrill of a ride.

Bring to Boil

Start by lighting candles all around the room. This is your *au naturel* swinging sex experience, so illuminate the room with natural light. If you have a fireplace, set up the swing in front of it in the winter months so you can both play nude and still keep warm by the heat of the flickering flames.

Get in the mood for motion by synching your body rhythms through dance. Choose a slow song at first so you can eroticize each other with swaying hips and twisting torsos. Slowly undress each other down to your underwear and continue to dance together. Many couples dance fully clothed, but it can be intensely sensual to dance skin on skin. She can enhance the ambience of this natural, animalistic play by revealing herself in animal-print lingerie. (He can also have leopard-print briefs on if he chooses to really embrace the role of King of the Jungle!)

Take off each other's remaining items of clothing and dance together fully nude. To switch from sensual to sexual, she can get him hard by taking him in her mouth to get him fired up. Once she's in the sex swing he will dictate most touch, so this is her main opportunity to give him pleasure under her control.

When you both start feeling hot for a swing-set session, she should move over to the swing and get in it. This may be difficult to do in a sexy, or even ladylike way, so she should abandon that idea and just hoist herself up into it butt first, legs in stirrups second (and he can help too). When she's comfortable, and all strapped in for the ride, he should spread her legs so they straddle each side of him. He can tickle her clitoris, finger her, and rub her wetness all over her lips and around the entrance to her vag so that penetration, thrusting in and all the way from the start, is made easy.

Swing her back and forth, guiding her along his shaft, rocking forwards and backwards. Create an easy momentum at first—a variety of slow and fast momenta are possible, without much effort. He will likely have to hold on to her, or the straps of the swing, to make sure she doesn't propel back too far and off of him. With a few practice thrusts they'll both get into the swing of it soon enough, so that when he pushes forward the swing moves back, and it will then naturally move back towards him again in its own motion.

Play with the versatility that the swing allows. She can squeeze her butt cheeks and splay her legs far to the side, to contain his penis from root to tip. She can then pulse her pelvic floor muscles to add rhythmic sensation for him (and for her). She can throw her head backwards and arch her back, which will automatically shift her hips upwards to engage him for a deep and tight sensation. Because all her body weight is supported by a suspension spring, he can easily bounce her up and down on him by placing his hands on her hips and circling her hips up, down and around him.

She can get a further rush by creating an inverse position, curling her head even further back so that her head drops, while he raises her legs to drop her head lower than her hips.

The blood will rush to her head and her vag muscles may twitch with this novel feeling.

With all the buoyancy the swing has, he can indulge his every desire to move her fast and hard against him without tiring too quickly. He should keep this furious motion short and sharp, though, because some women may not like it for long, and then make sure he stimulates her clit so that she regains her high arousal level. He can bring her to orgasm with his hand or a vibrator, which is easy for him to use on her since he's standing right over her with ready access. She might find that, even though all her weight is supported in the swing, she still needs to use her major muscles to remain balanced in the swing. This is good for her sexual response, because the more she uses her muscles, the greater the blood flow and the more likely she'll turn on her pelvic muscles, which will stimulate the sensitive tissue around her clitoris inside and out, helping to bring her to orgasm faster.

Both bob like mad until climax, with him using every conceivable twist of the swing to stimulate every angle of her vagina and each sensitive inch of his shaft. Now *that's* a rumble in the jungle—*schwiiing!*

Extra Zing
To add an extra dimension to your swinging loveplay, blindfold her so that when she's in the swing she becomes acutely aware of the sensation of being suspended in the air, and at the mercy of your touch, dictated to and controlled solely by you. As she spins and rocks in the dark, she won't know whether she's coming or going—but she will know when she cums . . .

Mud Cake

A sploshing good time.

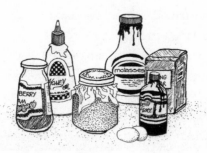

Pleasure Pantry Ingredients
A splash of this and a splosh of that:
  Oil
  Honey
  Jam
  Icing
  Yogurt
  Raw eggs
  Avocado
  Banana
  Strawberries
  Milk
  Oatmeal
  Pudding
  Custard
  Any other sticky, slimy food that tickles your fancy!

Plastic sheeting
Wading pool (optional)
Mud (optional)

Preparation
"Sploshing" is defined as erotic play with anything wet or messy, especially food. There are two main categories of

sploshing. The first is more mainstream, and allows couples to create a sexy mess together by indulging in food as tactile foreplay. The second is more exploratory, and involves becoming aroused through the wet sensations of smearing food all over each other—and the slipperier, messier, dirtier, more chaotic, the better.

Sploshing isn't everyone's cup of tea. In fact, most people would view it as really "out-there" extreme sex. Remember, though, that you can splosh a little or a lot—there are degrees of intensity when it comes to sexplay with food.

The emphasis when sploshing is on the slimy sensations of the various foods dribbling and trickling down your body, not the tasty ingestion of the actual ingredients—the combination of foods would make even the most cast-iron stomach turn. So this sexplay is a complete indulgence of *external* enjoyment.

Prepare for your unruly food sexplay by laying a large plastic sheet on the floor and arranging a buffet of foods and condiments around the outer edges for easy access. If ever you were going to let go and get down and dirty, this is the time.

Bring to Boil

Start your slippery good time by liberally dribbling oil over the plastic sheet to create a slick under-layer beneath you. Invite your lovee onto the pleasure place of prospective mess and then smear your hands slick with oil and stroke each other from tip to toe with the oil. This is a slow introduction to the potential of sexy slime because it's actually much like a massage, except the goal is distinctly different: a massage is light on oil and heavy on relaxation; sploshing is heavy on slippery, wet stimulation and very light on relaxation. The intention is to smoothly arouse rather than sedate.

If you've never played with food and sensual sex before, start with more traditionally erotic ingredients so that you can maintain and heighten a sense of arousal as you play with each other. Sit across from each other, close enough so that you're touching, and each reach over and feel for your first sensual ingredient, maybe something like honey or custard. Slop your fingers into it and then circle them around your partner's chest and down their belly. Take more and smear them with the substance across their shoulders and down their arms. Ask them to close their eyes as you continue, so they focus on the sense of touch rather than on the knowledge of what they're being touched with.

You may both be happy to play just enough to get slippery together all over before writhing horizontally in penetrative play. If you'd like to experiment further, though, amuse and arouse each other with more unusual foods that may not be traditionally sexy but can still deliver a wildly erotic sensation on the body. Peel a banana, orally suck it suggestively, then vehemently mash it and slime it all over your partner's groin and hips. You could crack an egg and then open it over their head, massaging their scalp and hair with the raw yolk and white. Pour milk down the outside of their throat and watch the white trickle weave its way down to their groin. Rub it in.

You can go to the extreme by taking viscous food, like oatmeal, and slop it over their chest or legs or shoulders. You may not think this is sexy—and for most people it's not—until you're in the middle of this kind of sploshing sexperimentation and you feel the absolute goo of thick oatmeal dribbling down your body. You may find its dense, skin-tingling sensation to be unlike any other, and the mess it creates liberating.

Sploshing is not serious, so have fun with it and each other. Delight each other with spontaneous sensations, and feel free to laugh at the imaginative ingredients and your random responses. Giggle at each other and at the feelings you experience. Laughter releases endorphins and decreases stress hormones in the body, so play of this kind can be viewed not only as a sensual experience but a de-stressing tonic.

When you're both suitably slimed and primed, lie side by side and face to face so both your bodies are still in contact with the slick plastic cover sheet. She can then bend down and lick his dick clean. It's important that his penis be as ingredient-free as possible before penetration, because foreign substances such as food can interfere with the natural flora of the vagina (it's always best to be as natural as possible after playing with food, or anything else, before you proceed to penetration, to protect the natural pH balance of the vagina). Once he's clean as a whistle—at least on his willy—generously go at it like you're famished for each other. Come cleanly amidst the sludge. Leave the rest of the cleaning for later.

Sploshing food sex may seem a chaotic mess, but it's good, clean fun.

Extra Zing

Take your slimy sploshing fun to a more passionate level of play by engaging in a mud wrestle together.

Set up an inflatable wading pool somewhere safe in your home, such as the laundry, garage, courtyard or back yard. Fill it with a vat of oil or lather it with pudding, or even the real thing—mud itself. Compete with each other in all-over body wrestling, the stakes being that the winner can claim the next sex encounter together, right down to their every whim.

Once you've prepped your wading pool, strip down to being completely naked—you don't want leverage advantages for the other through accessories such as ties or G-strings. Cake each other abundantly with your chosen ingredient, from top to bottom, to prepare an even playing field. Feel free to generously apply your chosen slick substance over their nether regions to distract them from their goal—be a strategic player! Men generally have more upper body strength than women, while ladies have greater lower body agility, flexibility and strength. However, the slipperiness of any slimy substance can quickly nullify any potential advantage. Wrestle with each other to try to pin your partner down. The one who can successfully dominate the other, in full body contact to the count of five, wins. The winner can then determine sex either right there and then, in the shower cleaning off, after the shower, or even negotiate a pleasure date further in the week or month. The winner takes all—of the other, in any which way they please, whenever they please.

Bottoms Up

Loving each other from top to bottom.

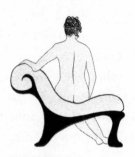

Pleasure Pantry Ingredients
Lube
G-string
Condoms (optional)
Vibrator (optional)
Anal vibrator (optional)
Anal beads (optional)
Anal dildo (optional)

Preparation

The backside is one of the last frontiers when it comes to sexual experimentation. Even though anal sex is ancient—lovers have been exploring the back door for thousands of years—it staunchly remains as one of our last taboos. Despite the large presence of anal loving in porn, in reality it's an activity a lot of couples haven't attempted—but are often curious about.

The excitement of trying a sexual taboo can make a couple feel naughty, "dirty," and even a bit fearful. Research shows, though, that there is a strong relationship between fear and pleasure. Feelings of fear are closely related to physical pleasure responses, and studies show that fearful feelings can sometimes be transposed to feelings of intense pleasure and desire. So if you're feeling fearful about trying anal sex, this can, to some degree, work in your favor because these fearful feelings can also create quickened blood-pumping to elicit arousal throughout your whole body, and especially in your nether regions (including your pelvic floor and anal area).

While a little bit of fear is okay, too much will shut down your sexual arousal. Some research indicates that fear can play a positive role in initial excitement, but as arousal increases make sure you engage in plenty of foreplay prior to penetration to maximize your pleasure nerves' response and settle your anxious nerves.

If you've never had anal sex, it can be helpful to decrease the anxiety around trying it by learning about the potential pleasure it can bring, so develop a bit of awareness of the vast network of pleasurable nerve endings present in the anus and anal canal. Both men and women have nerves which can be pleasingly stimulated in the anal area, and this is even truer for men, who can experience intense pleasure from a prostate massage up the bottom. Regardless of whether you're experimenting with anal sex with her or him, as receiver, there are some basic preparations you need to make the experience a pleasurable one.

You can opt to prepare for rear play by waxing (or shaving) for a smooth, sleek feel for you both. You can wax well before-hand, or shave each other as a primer to the event, but do so carefully so that you don't nick each other and so that your lube, when applied, doesn't sting. (Or you can simply skip this step and keep your back bush if that's your natural desire.)

Mentally eroticize the area by thinking of the anus and anal canal as an entrance to pleasure, rather than as an exit for other functions. The anus can be a very enticing introduction to a world of tight, titillating, taboo pleasure. Remember: the only filth you're channelling is erotic sexual experimentation. This positive mind connection is vital, because when it comes down to penetration, a positive, sexy association with that area of your body will help to relax you, which will also then increase your arousal and the sensations for you and your partner. If you and your partner have been flirting with the idea of "going there," this is now your opportunity to try a flirty, dirty poke from the rear.

Bring to Boil
She can wear her favorite G-string to show off her butt, provide a cheeky tease for him and to get her feeling like her whole derrière is super-sexy. Have lots of foreplay to get hot and horny as the more aroused she is, the more she'll be able to relax. Alternate anal arousal with clit stimulation by flicking and circling around her clit glans and then down around her perineum and along her anus. Pay attention to sensualizing the whole body and not just concentrating on the bum. Engage in lots of kissing and connecting through body, words and eyes so she doesn't feel pressured to go anal too soon, and so she doesn't feel disconnected from him: connection and trust are key ingredients to pleasurable anal play. Use lots and lots of lube—you cannot have too much. He should use it to stroke her up and down, and then up and down his shaft, and with one finger take a dollop of it and give her anus and bum crease a light, wet, tickling massage. Light touch here will flick on every single one of the many

nerves, and will physically show her just how sensitive this area of her body really is.

He needs to give her lots of kisses, and if he's using oral-friendly lube (bought at sex shops in different flavors), go down on her clit and lips, and then let his tongue travel even further southwards, and orally pleasure the sensitive spots just around her back hole.

With lots of lube on his fingers, he can slowly, very slowly, insert one finger up her bottom. If she tenses up, he should stop and let her adjust to the feeling of him being up there. He can curl his finger in a "come hither" motion to give her a slight extra sensation of being filled and tickled from the back. When she's comfortable, he can pull out and try adding a second finger in. He can then reach around and stimulate her clitoris so she remains aroused.

When you're both ready for the big event, situate yourselves so that he is sitting so she'll be able to lower herself onto him. This sitting position is ideal, but one least considered when couples visualize themselves having anal sex. This is because people often have a porn image of anal sex in the rear-entry position, with the man thrusting vigorously into the woman—any woman even the least bit hesitant about trying anal penetration can be scared off by this image.

The key to successful, pain-free initial anal penetration is to, first, allow the receiver to retain full control and, second, to lube up the penis and anus as much as possible. She can take a handful of lube and rub it up and down his shaft to really get the feel of the slickness about to go up and into her. If it's her first time, she can relax knowing that she is in control of the pace and depth. If the sitting position doesn't appeal, the woman-on-top (with him lying down) is also a good one; but if anything feels uncomfortable or painful, springing off is easier if she's on her feet, squatting over his lap, rather than on her knees sitting on him. Sitting, she can straddle his lap either facing him, or facing away.

Communicate with each other about when it feels good and when it feels too tight, or even when it hurts—which it shouldn't, really, and if it does then stop. (Important note: if you're not sure of your partner's full sexual history, or you're engaging in both vaginal and anal penetration, it's best to use a condom when you enter the rear.)

If anal play isn't new for you, but you'd like to add some more thrill for you both, hand over the control to the penetrating partner rather than the receiver. Thrusting doggy, porno style, can be wildly erotic for you both as she's plunged into at unpredictable depth and speed, and he dictates a rhythm of pleasure feeling acutely gripped tightly around his shaft as he slides in and out. To give both partners the ability to come, and come hard, place a vibrator against her clit. The pulses of her orgasm will make her whole bottom throb inside, and he'll relish every one of her happy tremors before he explodes too.

Extra Zing

Add some sizzle to your back-door play by giving him a prostate massage. The prostate is packed with pleasurable nerve endings, and can be reached by placing fingers up the butt. Move your finger(s) back and forth to massage this little secret sex organ, which can get a man so excited that he comes like never before. Some men find that the experience produces a "streaming" rather than "spurting" ejaculation, and swear that the sensation of orgasm is longer and more intense. Whether you choose to give a prostate massage by fingering him up the back, or with an anal vibrator, pulse against the prostate gland to elicit a streaming flow of orgasmic pleasure.

To increase playful experimentation in your anal loving, add toys! You can choose from a wide variety of toys in any sex shop or online sex outlet. There are anal beads, anal dildos (of all shapes, and the thin ones can be good in foreplay if either partner is a bit nervous about larger, thicker penetration) and anal vibes. When playing from the back—his or hers—remember: safety first. Experiment, but only with good, clean toys especially designed for back use. Play well, and you'll both want to go back . . . for more.

Quick & Easy

Why want love
lust was
always
tremendously
satisfying

Sweet Chilli Eve

Pre-party passion

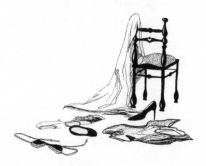

Pleasure Pantry Ingredients
15 extra minutes

Preparation

Spice up your evening with a red-hot root before you go out—the memory will stay with you all night and you'll smile your way through your dinner party or evening work function.

This is all about desire—wanting each other so badly that you need to screw before you head out for the evening. You simply can't wait, and want to have each other sooner rather than later. Most evenings, couples who get ready to go out put effort into dressing up, looking sexy and smelling nice, and then they throw on their coats and head out. They look their best only to spend the evening socializing with others. Then, at the very end of the night, maybe they'll make love when they get home—if they're not too over it to get into it.

For this evening, give yourselves to each other when you're both looking your most desirable—before you even go out. If you have each other now, you'll want each other all night, and the electricity between you will flicker continuously.

There is no preparation needed for pre-party passion except a little extra time to squeeze in a quickie. Or not. You could just say 'screw it' and arrive 15 minutes fashionably late and unfashionably flushed.

Bring to Boil

Use the power of the skirt. Men love reaching up under skirts, getting a glimpse of what you're wearing underneath and taking a forbidden touch. Ask him if he likes what you're wearing. Lift up your skirt and ask him again if he likes what you're wearing. Do this with an inviting, teasing attitude. It won't take much to give him the idea, and you won't have to ask twice.

A lot of women might avoid the pre-function fuck because they've put time and energy into looking good and don't want to mess up their face, clothes or lipstick. So he might be surprised that you want to reverse the norm and this can give you a powerful charge that turns you on even more. Create a quickie that's all about harried, have-to-have-you-now sex, and forget about the romantic kissing and canoodling. Leave that for another evening, or later in the night when you're home and can take more time. It can be intensely erotic to throw caution and sensibility aside and have sex simply because you want to, because you want to smell and feel your partner's sexy scent on you all night. This kind of quickie serves as a primer, not the night's peak.

Pull up your skirt and reveal your sexy underwear to your partner. With him watching, slide your hand down the front of your panties and get a good feel of your own wetness. Then take his hand and wipe your fingers inside his palm. Pull his hand down to your undies and invite him to take them off. Grind your hips from side to side as an invitation, not that he'll need it. Bend over the dressing table and let him take you from behind. Once he's penetrated you, shift your legs close together and squeeze your pelvic floor muscles for an extra snug fit as he slides in and out of you. This muscle tensing can heighten the sensations for you, too, and if the sex isn't too quick you might rise to orgasm, or near to it.

If your dressing table has a mirror, take in the view. Watch him fuck you in your outfit; look at him, fully dressed, plunging into you. Cement an image of this in your mind— each of you—so you can recall it throughout the evening to really get you both hot under the collar all night.

Extra Zing

Keep your panties off and at opportune (or inopportune) moments, let your partner feel that you've got your panties off . . . a sexy taunt for round two, later! The first feel-up could be in the car, or discreetly in the cab, right before you arrive. A touch, a wink and a smile is all it takes to make them rethink the whole evening and want to turn around and head straight home and into bed. But prolonging the anticipation will make the evening a spicy one, because you'll be immensely sexually attracted to each other all evening, sharing a secret across the room, without even touching.

Just before you enter your destination, reach over and tell your partner that you've hidden your panties somewhere at home, and you won't have sex with him again until he finds them. This really ups the sexual tension because he'll go crazy trying to think where they might be, titillated by the sexy hide-and-seek game to come and frustrated that the playing has to wait. The evening will loom ahead, but every time you look at each other you can recall the image of fucking, fully dressed, just as you are, only a little while ago. He'll remember the panties you had on—the very ones he slid down your legs, from under your skirt—and be every inch aware that you do not have them on now, and that they're hiding, somewhere—not here—waiting to be found, to serve as the permission to have you again.

When you do get home, draw out the flirty game by playing strip sexual hide-and-seek. Each time he gets warmer, take off an item of your outfit. If he gets colder, put it back on. Because men are visual, these cues will propel his search with even more fervour. When he does find your undies, heating up the rest of your sweet chilli night is up to you . . .

Smells Like Sex and Candy

Sex for dessert—sweeten your night with honeyed-up loving.

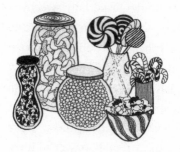

Pleasure Pantry Ingredients
Scented candles
Honey
Powdered sugar
Package of peppermints (optional)

Preparation
Get in the mood for sugary lovemaking by creating an ambience of sweet sensuality. Not all quickies have to occur without a little attention to detail, so have some fun making each other irresistible to touch, suck, lick and love.

The key to sex as dessert is to remember that both men and women report wishing that they had time for more sex in their lives, so sometimes satisfying sex isn't necessarily about a long lovemaking session, but more about making a short time a good time. Quickies have earned a bad reputation as sex that can't be satisfying, simply because it's quick. The average length of intercourse is 10 minutes—that doesn't sound much, until you think about how much pleasure can actually be concentrated into 10 minutes!

Bring to Boil

You can enhance the experience by illuminating your sex-play with a few candles, especially sweetly scented ones that will complement the aromatic aura created by dribbling honey over each other. Choose a scented candle that reminds you of each other, or of an erotic memory you share. For example, you may have taken a beach vacation together and spent every day making love in the heat. Lighting a coconut-scented candle will bring back those memories, especially because smell is an extremely powerful memory trigger, and you can fantasize and channel those erotic feelings to rapidly escalate your arousal and desire for each other.

Undress your partner and lay them down on a washable blanket, spread out over the bed. Or simply say 'fuck it' and do it directly on the bed, knowing that having to wash honey off the sheets later will be worth it.

Using a spoon or honey dribbler, drip honey slowly over their chest and nipples. A little goes a long way, and you don't want to get sick licking it off or make too much of a sticky mess ... yet. Occasionally put a little honey on your finger and trace your partner's lips with it, to give them a little sweet taste which can sensually stimulate them to close their eyes and concentrate on taste and touch. Using alter-nating quick flicks of your tongue and hot, flat licks, trace the honey trail down past their navel. Dab a small dollop of honey on their glans and spread it around with your warm, wet fingers. Both the glans of the clitoris and of the penis are populated with nerve endings, so paying attention directly to this area will bring about orgasm faster. However, one of the main mistakes of couples who indulge in quickies is to plunge into penetration too soon, and this hinders the chance of the woman being able to come.

Tease your partner with more lingering sweetness by adding some visual sugar to your lovemaking—lick your fingers and coat them in powdered sugar. Suck your partner's sticky, honeyed nipples and sprinkle them with more powdered sugar. Heightening arousal by bringing your partner right to the edge through plenty of short but intense manual and oral play, using one or two extras like a bit of sugar, will intensify the desire to have intercourse so that when you do it will be explosive, both physically and mentally. It won't last long, but that's the point!

The preferred position by most couples who enjoy quickies is the man-on-top. Add a little variation to this by having her swing her legs over his shoulders to allow for deep penetration. The deep penetration will enable him to come super-quickly because each thrust is receiving maximum length, warmth and tight stimulation. She can continue the visual feast by licking or sucking her own honey- and powdered-sugar-coated fingers while staring him straight in the eyes with smoldering enjoyment directed squarely at him. He'll burst.

Extra Zing

For an extra tantalizing tingle for you—and him—play with peppermint candies. Suck on a peppermint in your mouth, then take it out and roll it down your torso before tucking it between your lower lips at the entrance to your vagina. Then invite him to suck it out. Encourage him to roll it over your mound and between your lips, over your clitoral hood and up the clitoral shaft, and then lick everywhere he rolled the mint. He could also blow on your skin to give a cool, tingling feeling. Many people will respond to the slight menthol sensation of the mint, so it's important not to use mints that are too strong in case you're sensitive and it burns slightly.

You can also take this quickie fantasy one step further by embodying the sex-and-candy theme with your clothes. She might put on a pair of colorful candy-striped knee-high socks and pair it with hot red stilettos. He might leave his shirt on, open and stained with honey and sugar. Go for it with a mirror to the side of you, so you can both watch. Yum.

With your boudoir smelling of sweet dessert sex, hop under the sheets and go to bed. Who says there wasn't time for a fun quickie at night? And isn't it more lip-smackingly delicious than TV and a Toblerone?

Espresso Morning

Coffee and a quickie—give your heart a shot of energy by starting the day with a hot hit!

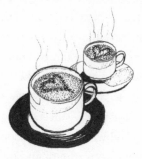

Pleasure Pantry Ingredients
Alarm clock
Coffee

Preparation

Most men would, if they could, start their day with an orgasm. Especially one brought about by their lover. His Morning Glory is his hardest erection, and the orgasm he feels from its release is explosively powerful. Whether or not your man pesters you for morning sex, on this particular morning you're going to give him—and you—a full-strength erotic energizer.

If you set your alarm early and get up to put the coffee on (unless you have a timer coffee percolator that automatically switches on in the morning), you can surprise your partner with coffee, and you, in bed.

Bring to Boil

Appear in the bedroom doorway with two cups of coffee. Topless. You might still be wearing pyjama bottoms, or you might have put on some lingerie. The sight of you will give him an endorphin-rush brain snap, because he might be unused to seeing you in sexy lingerie in the morning, sexily flaunting your breasts above two steaming cups of hot coffee, that smell of both "wake up" and "home."

Coffee has a powerful aroma, so take a sip and give him a kiss; then, after your second sip and while your mouth is still hot from the coffee and you're still standing on the side of the bed, bend over him and wrap your lips around the head of his penis so it's just inside your mouth and on your tongue, and put your warm coffee taste all over his head and shaft. Let him watch you bend over him for a few licks and sucks, so he can take in the sight of your mouth going up and down on him, and your breasts swaying with the rhythm you create.

Then pull the sheets down past his ankles and climb onto the bed with him. Let him continue to watch you take control of his body and sexual response. A lot of couples who have morning sex don't kiss (morning breath), don't open their eyes (fantasies prevail over the sight of sleepy faces and slept-on hair), and hide under the covers in the light of day. This morning, though, the combination of caffeine and being able to relax and feel and watch you will charge him up for a pumping good start to the day.

When he is groaning with pleasure from watching you go down on him, climb on top and straddle him, but don't let him enter you yet. Arch up and drop one of your nipples into his mouth. Circle your breasts over his face, drawing attention to them. Take one of his hands and guide him to your clit. Think of your clit as a coffee bean, compact but brimming with contained energy. Tell him you're going to come before he can enter you, and tell him you want to come fast. But you stay in control of the pace and pressure—don't let go of his hand. The excitement here is that its usually men who have a morning wank. What you're doing is letting him in on your morning wank, while you sit on him. Tell him just about when you're going to come and, as you do, put his fingers inside of you. He should be positively frothing by now, so shift back and slide on top of him.

The woman-on-top position is one of the best for the first morning erection, precisely because his penis is so hard. Sometimes with a softer erection women can, through the swivelling of their hips, bend the penis into slight discomfort (or extreme pain if she pulls up too high and then bangs her body weight back down on him, which can be a common misjudgment). With the stiff morning erection, it's usually easier for her to really ride him, hard and fast. This is, after all, a hot morning quickie.

If your man is a breast man, face him as you ride him. If he's a butt guy, turn around and ride him facing his feet, so he can get a good view of your bum cheeks separated and sliding up and down his shaft. After he comes, lean over to his face, give him a kiss, whisper "good morning," get off him, reach for your coffee cup, and walk naked out of the bedroom and into the shower. Give him a moment alone to ponder on how he got so lucky!

Extra Zing
To really get his blood pumping, consider giving him a quick handless massage using your hair, lips, teeth, elbows,

legs, face and, yes, breasts to invigorate him awake. You can incorporate these alternating sensations between teasing coffee-mouth penis kisses and sucks.

To add a bit of extra sensation when you're riding him, try the technique of "milking the penis." Squeeze your pelvic floor muscles each time you ride him up, then relax them as you slide back down his shaft, then pulse them. Work yourself into a rhythm that feels good to you—and it might even help to think about the technique as a "milking." Once you're comfortable with that, try it swivelling your hips from side to side as you go up and down. If this is all too much focus for an early-morning quickie, don't worry—he's already blown away by you.

Why go out for Starbucks when you've got starfucks at home?

Root 69

Driver reviver! The car quickie.

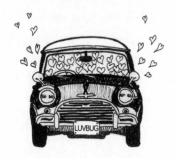

Pleasure Pantry Ingredients
Car
A secluded spot

Preparation

Most men love cars. And they like bonking in cars. Before we had houses of our own we played in cars, so having a quickie in a car takes us back to those fumbling but exciting adolescent experiences of making out in the back of a car, or even just pashing in the front seat. The idea of having sex in the car, somewhere in public, brings with it the thrill of doing something a bit naughty, of perhaps getting caught, and that sense of risk increases the heart rate and thus blood flow in the body—especially down to the genitals. This increased blood flow creates fast and hard erections in a man, and for a woman's clitoris too, and sparks a twitching anticipation, a yearning to accelerate to touching each other naked.

If you're on a road trip, heighten the anticipation by playing a little "I like" game. Each time you see a sign indicating how many miles to your destination, each of you must say to the other something that you like them to do to you. This not only puts sex firmly on the agenda, it's a great way to get your partner to reveal to you things they really like you to do to them sexually, and you can bear these in mind when you finally do arrive and check in. In the meantime, as you're heating up for a car quickie, each of you can reflect on the tips you're sharing and start visualizing doing them to each other. You'll be steaming up the windows with your sex talk before you even pull over for your quickie!

Bring to Boil

It's important to find a secluded spot when you pull off the road for your quickie—it is most definitely illegal to be seen having sex in public, and as exciting as the risk of getting caught is, actually being caught can put a serious dampener on your sexual experience.

Many people become frustrated trying to have sex in a car because it is a little bit like playing Twister for two in a cramped, awkward space. There are a few options, however, the consensus seems to be that the best position is indeed in the back seat—but sitting up, rather than both trying to squeeze in horizontally, with heads bumping and feet leaving pressed footprints into the car ceiling. He should be seated in the middle of the back seat, and she can sit on his lap, either facing him or facing away. A benefit of facing him is that you're both looking in opposite directions, so, should someone approach the car, one of you will notice. That is, if you can see out of the steamed windows!

In order to enhance the thrilling perception of potentially getting caught, and to keep things moving, don't bother getting undressed. The car quickie is a classic for tops wrapped around necks and pants twirled around ankles.

To make the car quickie exhilarating, especially for her, and to escalate the arousal beyond a short-relief bonk, he needs to instil some confidence in her ability to drive him wild while she's on top of him, in the squashed back seat—so he should give her plenty of stimulating attention. The kind of attention he gives his beloved car. He can buff her body with circular motions that show her his need and desire for her. And suck her nipples until they are hard headlights. Reach down and polish her clit as she rides him—he's got perfect access because she's right on top of him in close quarters.

As she's moving on him, and he's giving her erogenous zones a good gloss, he can think of his—and her—sexual response as a finely tuned motor, and vary the speed. He may put a hand on her hip and drive her rhythm up and down. Or really rev it up by going fast and furious, but vary the gears by slowing down and then shifting it into high and hard again. Both the female and male sexual responses have several arousal gears, and the pleasure plateau before orgasm is when you can really modify the pace to fuel those fulfilling sensations.

While men are more visual, women respond to auditory stimulation (as long as she likes what he's saying), so he can make her really purr with passion by sharing his appreciation for how well-built she is, how he loves her curves, how fantastic she feels holding his dick inside her.

You can make noise in a car, especially in a secluded spot, because in the car you're isolated together, completely alone in your own space. So talk, grunt, growl, groan—express your urges.

When it's done, if she hasn't come because he was slightly distracted from her clit by her amazing shaft-shifting techniques on him, he should reach down and kick into manual gear to hot-wire her to orgasm. Just as he would feel pain from trapped blood flow in his penis, after all that excitement, if he didn't orgasm, she'll be in a similar state of pain if she doesn't also experience a release—not a good adolescent memory to emulate in this instance. And just because the car is small, and the sex is quick, that's no excuse not to both race to the finish line.

Extra Zing

The 69 position is not the most elegant at the best of times, and certainly requires some contortionist moves in a car. However, if you want to add a bit of saucy naughtiness to your sexplay in the car, try to mutually satisfy each other orally rather than manually. You can try to entwine horizontally in the back seat but, really, the best type of car for this particular activity is, of course, the shaggin' wagon.

Because the risk of getting caught is even higher with 69 than with a backseat rumble (eyes are most definitely not on the road while 69'ing!), keeping most of your clothes on is a smart strategic move.

The car quickie isn't about sensual, quality lovemaking. It's wicked and fun and a release. If you want to draw out your sexplay in the car—especially if you're on a long driving trip—at every third Driver Reviver pit stop, sneak off and take turns pleasing and playing with each other, until you're maxed out and on empty—and in need of a different kind of Driver Reviver!

Wash-n-Go

A classic—the shower quickie.

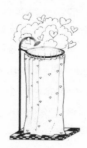

Pleasure Pantry Ingredients
Shower accessories: shampoo, conditioner, loofah, soap
Oil, preferably scented
"Rubber Dickie" (optional)

Preparation
Hop in the shower with your partner!

Couples who shower together, especially in the morning, find it to be a happy expression of their union before getting on with their day. While a night shower together can be just as sexy, the morning is usually better because energy levels are higher, as are testosterone levels—both critical ingredients for a quickie.

Have an extra 15 minutes to spare, as shower quickies are "quick" compared to other sexual indulgences but usually make for a longer-than-normal shower.

Bring to Boil
Take turns lathering each other up and down. Shampoo each other's hair, giving a good scalp massage to invigorate them

and make them tingle from the top down. Then use the slip-periness of the lather to begin teasing handiwork on your partner's nether regions. Really concentrate on how erotic your partner's skin feels under your wet, slick touch.

Now rinse, kiss, and reach for the oil. Pour a little oil across your partner's shoulders, and into your palms, and start to work in from the shoulders down. Knead with your fingers and the heel of your hand. Give them deep, long strokes, not only to relax them with a massage—mimicking the strokes of penetration stimulates the mind and heightens the pace of desire. Be careful not to use too much oil, though, because you'll need grip for leverage in less than five minutes.

Many people like to kiss, suck and lick their partner as they share a shower, particularly if they are sensitive to their partner's taste and smell, and don't feel comfortable giving or receiving oral sex in general. Shower sex is a good way to indulge in oral stimulation because the cascade of water washes over you, and them, and they may even be steaming with the smell from the scented oil you're using. Scented oil is preferable to unscented because, as it is absorbed into the skin, it will serve as a reminder all day (or all night) of the erotic experience you shared. This sensual memento fuels libido throughout the day because it keeps sex on your brain—and a smile on your face.

When your desire for each other is ravenous, shift from oiling each other's pleasure zones to intercourse in the standing position. Most showers require some creative manoeuvring to comfortably fit two partners at the right height and accessibility for penetration. If your shower is in a tub, use the edge of the tub for height leverage. Put a towel down on the edge of the tub to lean your weight on, as opposed to slipping on the porcelain (especially with feet that have been slathered with oil). If you still find this difficult, as many couples do, have him sit on the towel on the edge of the tub, where she can straddle him, either facing him or facing away. This position is excellent because it dispenses with the height, weight and leverage issue, and can allow for the quickie to go just a bit longer, as each partner's weight is supported.

If your shower is a standard one, frankly there are really only two primary position options: quick and quicker. For the quicker position, he can hold her weight up entirely, with her legs wrapped around him, drawing him deeply into her. Holding all his partner's weight will mean he's engaging most major muscle groups and he will come quickly. Less intensive (and often far more practical) is the standing position in which he lifts and holds one of her legs to open her hips, and penetrates with a bending (knee trembling!) motion. She can hang on to him with her arms, or, if she is a similar height to him, she can help dictate the rhythm by holding her hands on his hips.

If the standing position in the shower proves too difficult to pull off successfully, you're not alone. Many couples avoid sex in the shower because it can be so tricky. Successful shower sex can simply mean having an erotic feel-up together, before fumbling out of the shower and onto a pile of towels in the bathroom, or finishing with hot, wet, slithering intercourse, sliding together onto the bed.

Once you're done, kiss and towel each other and later, during the day, each time you get a whiff of the scent of the oil on your skin, take a moment to remember your morning and feel again the arousal you bring to each other.

Extra Zing

For that extra stimulation, especially for her, use a water-safe toy to stimulate her clitoris. While women regularly enjoy quickie sex without orgasm, it can be frustrating when the sex is particularly erotic, as a good shower quickie can be with that all-over body teasing and slippery hand stimulation. Because the water in a shower can quickly wash away her natural lubrication, if you do use a water-safe vibrating toy on her vulva during the shower quickie, be sure to add lubrication. The best lubricant to use is a specially designed lube for sex toys, so you know it won't interfere with the material the toy is made of—but this is really up to you. Share the toy on each other's bodies, liberally stimulating her clitoris, his and her nipples and inner thighs, as well as the shaft of his penis. A recommended toy is the "Rubber Dickie." This toy looks and feels like the ideal shower quickie accessory, and can be bought at most adult shops or online sex boutiques.

If you'd rather not use a water-safe sex toy, or don't have one, a removable shower head is just as effective. Massage it into her inner lips and clitoris, using the pressure of the water to create a motion that will have her hips grinding and gliding in delight!

Chance Encounter

Seize the sex—the opportunity quickie.

Pleasure Pantry Ingredients
Absolutely nothing—work with what you've got in the heat of the moment.

Preparation
Having sex by seizing the moment can be wildly erotic, mostly because engaging in sex at the "wrong" time can feel oh so right. Fortune quickies heighten the sense of desire between lovers because chance encounters are at the opposite end of the spectrum from "routine sex": they are unpredictable and spontaneous. This makes them h-o-t and they require no preparation at all.

Bring to Boil
Chance encounters can have the fantasy feel of a random experience with a stranger. You can capture the feel of a clandestine one-night stand while being with your regular partner because the essence of the sexual high comes from how spectacularly inappropriate the act is at that particular time and

place. Opportunity quickies can occur in the most unexpected and seemingly unsexy locations: at your nan's eighty-third birthday party; on your office desk while a work function buzzes in the staff room; at weddings and family get-togethers; in back-yard corners and alleyways, and those opportunities which seem too good to be true—those obvious disappearances where you think you're getting away with sneaking off to the bathroom together but you're really not.

Thinking that someone may discover you and be outraged can make a shared secret session feel as intense as an illicit affair, without the guilt. When you indulge in a chance encounter with each other, the sex is selfish and unseemly—but you just can't help yourselves. You shouldn't do it, and that's why you love it. You feel filthy, but in a mischievously good way.

If you're lucky enough to find yourselves in a chance encounter where there's a bed (a spare room perhaps), then go ahead and bonk like bunnies, dust yourselves off, unrumple your clothes, and resurface like nothing's happened, except for the big fat smiles on your faces. Mostly, though, opportunity sex occurs in places that encourage up-against-the-wall sex. In loos, closets, and dark and (seemingly) secret corners, opportunity sex requires easy access and hasty humping.

Slipping off to have a sneaky quickie without being caught requires muscle control and smart positioning. Penetrate from the rear so she is facing away from him, holding on to the fence, back of the door or towel rack, or literally bending up against the wall. The lack of face-to-face contact heightens the randomness of the encounter, and also makes the rear-entry standing position—the least often used or preferred sexual position—a little easier because the man is not required to hold his partner's weight. She can arch her back, showing off her bootyliciousness, while also encouraging deeper penetration. If more connectedness is desired, he can press his whole torso against her back and grip her around her waist, or grab her wrists with his hands and stretch them above her head, so that full upper-body contact is achieved. Payoff: raw heat. Price tag: expect the odd bruise, especially if you're going hard. This kind of wild quickie embodies the concrete need to possess one another, at all costs, in any way possible, and the sense of the inability to resist each other, no matter how unsuitable the setting, is a powerful, unparalleled aphrodisiac.

Covert coupling will also require stealth and silence: the art of noise restraint should be applied. Suppress your sex sounds by biting on your partner's clothes, sucking their fingers or giving hickeys. Hickeys are about ownership and serve as sex trophies: proof positive that you were together, and that you've left your mark. They are skin stains of sex that you'll have with you for at least the next week, so don't blush or brag—just see it and remember.

Extra Zing

If you want to save opportunity sex for a truly different experience, wait until you take your next flight together as a couple and join the Mile High Club. A lot of couples toy with the idea of joining the ranks of those who have had soaring sex, but only a minority go through with it. After all, it takes a bit of preparation to successfully score at 30,000-plus feet.

First, wear loose clothing and only one layer—simplicity of entry is critical. The average jumbo jet toilet dimensions are 3 feet by 4 feet, so sex in the airline bathroom is essentially a wriggling lap dance. If he sits on the toilet and she sits on his lap, facing away, and leans her arm on the sink for leverage, two people can fit fairly comfortably. Otherwise, you can fit sideways in the cubicle: he can stand, and she can bend as far forward as possible, leaning over the sink; or, if there's a baby-changing table, that can be an even better option. On any flight, no matter how long, there is always going to be a line for the toilet every few minutes, so joining the Mile High Club is a rite of passage rather than a route of pleasure. He might climax, but she might have to finish herself off by returning to the bathroom alone a few minutes later. Regardless, the enjoyment of the escapade is in the novelty of it, so emerge in full smirk. You've earned your elite place among the sexual top guns.

Sweet

It's the touch
of your hand,
the warmth of
your breath
on my skin,
the yearning
your fingers stroke
out of me
that remind me
why I am here
and why I
stay

The Bedroom Picnic

A succulent lovers' picnic in the great indoors.

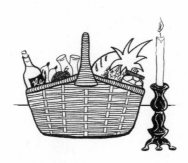

Pleasure Pantry Ingredients
Picnic basket set for two
Perfume/incense
Music/CD player
Candles—at least twenty
Soft blanket
Laminated love notes (optional)

Your sexy menu can contain the following aphrodisiac items:
Avocados
Almonds
Caviar
Prawns
Oysters
Tuna
Broccoli
Pumpkin
Eggs
Lentils
Beets
Tomatoes
Mushrooms
Truffles

Ginger
Basil
Cheese
Figs
Mangoes
Blackberries
Raspberries
Strawberries
Papayas
Bananas
Whipped cream
Chocolate
Wine/Champagne
Dessert liqueur

While the above items have been researched and found to contain a healthy number of vitamins, minerals and amino acids to boost desire and sexual function (even the alcohol, which acts as a relaxant and sexual disinhibitor, and has been shown to stimulate testosterone levels in small doses), you can substitute or add any other ingredients that take your fancy!

Preparation

A little attention and care to prepare your bedroom picnic will go a long way, because it will show your lovee that you are invested in nurturing the sexy side of your relationship. And the effort you go to will be richly rewarded!

The Bedroom Picnic is ideal for cold winter nights and wet-weather eves, or even hot summer nights when you can open your bedroom windows to let the summer breeze in while you enjoy each other in the comfort of your bedroom. A bedroom picnic revitalizes your bedroom as a place of seduction, flirtation and even dating, and not just a room in which you sleep and make love. The new context of your bedroom as a place where you romance and play will create memories that will last long after the picnic basket is packed away and the candles blown out.

To prepare for the Bedroom Picnic, pick a night when you can be alone in the house without distractions or looming work deadlines, so you can both relax. Get your picnic set ready and prepare your menu using at least some of the aphrodisiac items from the ingredients list. Prepare a cooler by the bed so that you can keep necessary items like wine or champagne cool during the evening. You may choose to make your own food, get takeaway, or a combination of both.

Earlier in the day, or even earlier in the week, invite your lovee to a special night in, but give no hints as to what the evening will entail. Let it be a surprise.

Just before your lovee is due to arrive home, make sure the bedroom is all set up. Lightly spritz the bedroom pillows with perfume or, if you prefer, light some incense to create a completely sensual experience. Put some music on low volume. Light candles all around the room, using twenty or more, to create a romantic atmosphere that is also light enough to see each other and the picnic spread. Arrange the soft blanket over the bed (to create a fresh setting to sit on, rather than your "regular" bed sheets, and to protect your doona covering from any potential stains or mess). Place the picnic basket up near the pillows and open it, revealing some of the goodies inside. Set the wine or champagne (or other beverage) in a cooler on the bedside table.

Bring to Boil
When your lovee arrives, greet them at the door with a kiss and a smile, and ask them if they're ready for their surprise.

If they need a moment or two after arriving to unwind from work (unless it's a sexy Saturday night, of course), allow them to do this—because you want their full attention once they enter the bedroom. Once they're relaxed, they can enjoy the total experience of the bedroom picnic with you.

Lead your partner into the bedroom, invite them to sit on the bed and pour them a drink. Clink glasses and toast your lovee with either a loving and heartfelt sentiment, or a frisky, playful comment.

Start your sexy feast slowly, with your appetisers to warm up, before proceeding to your main course. Feed each other. Make flirtatious satisfied noises. Talk and really take the time out to connect as a couple, without any distractions from work, children, TV, bills, family or domestic issues.

When you're ready for dessert, start with one sweet thing, such as berries. But before feeding your lover the sweetness, eat one seductively and smear some of the juice on your chin and neck, and take a hand to wipe it off, then smear the juice on their lips. Kiss the juice off them. As you kiss, take their top off and then take your own top off (if you haven't already done so) to give the strong hint that dessert entails more than just eating the food.

Using your chosen sweet dessert items (including fruit, chocolate and whipped cream), indulge in eating off each other's bodies. Take a raspberry and squeeze it over a nipple. Dribble whipped cream down their belly and lick it off. Once you've made yourselves wet and wildly messy on your top halves, undress each other until you're both completely nude. Continue your sweet indulgence on and with each other right down into each other's nether regions. Smear whipped cream between her lower lips and lick them clean.

Rub juice along his shaft and suck him like he's never tasted so good to you before. When the delectable deliciousness is coursing through you both, and you have to have more, put your arms around each other and, sitting up, make love in the oh-so-yummy Yab Yum position, which essentially has her sitting in his lap with her legs wrapped around and behind him. This is a Tantric sex position designed to connect both partner's bodies and draw out the sexual response so you can make love longer.

Using swivelling and grinding motions, maximize the intensity of the sensations by matching faster and harder rhythms, or slow down your arousal by decreasing the pace and the fervor of the pushing and grinding. Either partner can reach down and rub the clitoris, allowing her to come first or, timed between the two of you, to come at the same time.

When pleasurably replete, untwine yourselves and bask in the afterglow together, still by the light of the candles. You might like to enjoy a liqueur, and a rest, and then indulge in another course . . . of each other.

Extra Zing

To add even more passion to your picnic, create some homemade sexy "fortune cookies." Hand write, in red ink, some teasing and pleasing "fortunes" and laminate the paper so you can cut each of them into plastic protected strips. Attach one to each piece of chocolate, or chocolate cookie, tied with a small red ribbon in a bow, or cut some small indentations into the strawberries and insert a fortune into each one.

Your sexy fortunes might be miniature love notes, or they might be enticing suggestions such as, "You will be ravished by your lover from tip to toe," "Your lover will hunger for you tonight," "You will be loved and satisfied by your lover in every way you want tonight" and "Sex for dessert? Yes, and tonight you get extra helpings." Make up your own to suit your own tastes and then share the goodness between the both of you, handing the sexy "fortune cookies" to each other one by one. A sexy fortune, guaranteed to be good. Very, very good.

Vanilla Essence

Pure passion

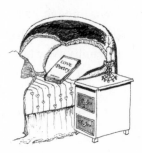

Pleasure Pantry Ingredients
Dinner reservations
Vanilla ice cream
Vanilla-scented candle
Book of love poems
Music
White satin and lace teddy lingerie
Engraved stationery (optional)
Wood and carving knife (optional)

Preparation

Capturing the essence of vanilla sex means enveloping your-selves in traditional romance and love. "Vanilla sex" refers to the most traditional lovemaking, without wild experimenta-tion. Some people think of vanilla sex as bland, but a better way of looking at it is simply lovely. And while it may not be heavy on spice, it's still got a lot of spark.

Couples often feel so much pressure to have hot, naughty sex all the time that they may go ages without reverting to one of the loveliest lovemaking experiences of them all: the nice time. Nice is good. Nice is sweet.

Interestingly, vanilla, while connoting "mild" and carrying with it the associations of "white," "pure" and even "virginal," actually has a stimulating effect on libido. Vanilla is considered by many to be an aphrodisiac because it acts on the central nervous system through its smell and taste, and produces an enhancing effect on sexual stimulation. So just because your sex may be vanilla, your lovemaking can still be creamy, smooth and, in essence, exquisitely enchanting.

Prepare for this experience by making dinner reservations at a sentimental restaurant. It might be where you had your first date, where you became engaged, or a place you both love. Make sure you have vanilla ice cream at home and one vanilla-scented candle in the bedroom on the bedside table, along with a favorite book of love poems. Leave the rest to romance.

Bring to Boil

Dress up to go out tonight; look special and feel special. When you arrive at the restaurant, choose valet parking if it's available. When you get to your table, he should try to head the maître d' off at the pass and pull the chair out for his lovee himself. Start the evening date by ordering a blushing champagne cocktail for you both. Then share some white wine as you dine on the traditional fare of lobster thermidor for two. Spend your dinner date talking and enjoying each other's company. This is a night of romance, so taboo conversation topics include: finances, children, work, worries or stressful subjects.

Make this a dreamy date. Talk about your hopes and dreams. Fantasize about your future together. Make a dream list of things you'd like to do as a couple, like buying a boat or boutique B & B, going on a trip across Europe or trekking across the snow-capped Himalayas, designing your dream home or taking a year off work to just play and read every book on your ultimate wish list. Whatever your dreams, they're yours to own and share tonight.

When your dinner date is over, and the bill paid, he should excuse himself to go and get the car (if valet parking wasn't available when you arrived), so he can drive it right up to the front of the restaurant to pick her up and save her walking in her heels across the parking lot, as a charming gesture of old-school romance. When he arrives in the car, he should—in traditional style—hop out and open the car door for her. Such seemingly small gestures of romance often dissipate, if not disappear, from long-term relationships, so on a night like tonight embrace every romantic tradition to create an atmosphere of loving attention and courtship.

Once home, light the scented candle in the bedroom and put on some quiet romantic music for background ambience. She can change into "something more comfortable" and join him in the bedroom wearing her brand-new satin and lace teddy lingerie.

By the light of the one flickering flame of the vanilla candle, make sweet love to each other as if discovering each other's bodies for the first time. Kiss your lovee from face to feet. Spend lots of time kissing on the lips, as if you were making out for the very first time. Make love in the traditional missionary position, with only one twist: making sure she has an orgasm too. It can be difficult for a woman to experience orgasm in the man-on-top position, so extra effort to stimulate her clitoris should be generously applied.

Bask in the loving afterglow of this wonderful vanilla sex, spending a little more romantic time together in bed before sleeping. Add sweetness by indulging in some vanilla ice cream together for a late-night dessert snack. One of you can get it from the kitchen, place two scoops in one bowl with a small dessert spoon and feed each other in bed. Eat, kiss, talk, laugh and share. Reach for the book of love poems; flick through so each of you can choose ones you like best. Read your favorites to each other out loud. Then snuggle down into the spoon position and fall asleep to the rhythm of each other's breaths and chests rising and falling against each other. Lovely. Memorable. And very nice.

Extra Zing

For some special added romance to your evening, prepare a romantic gift for one another. She can order him some engraved stationery with his name embossed on it. Writing notes by hand is a dying art, but with fine personalized stationery at his disposal, he may be more inclined to write letters, and to write you love notes.

Before wrapping the stationery, write a love poem to him—an ode to your love—and leave it at the top of the stack. If you don't feel that you are adept at writing love poetry, either transcribe a love poem you adore and share it with him, or simply write a list of words to describe why you love him, and love being with him, but set the words out on the page in a staggered fashion so it looks artistic and poetic.

For his gift he can purchase a piece of wood and carve a large love heart, and then carve his initials plus hers into the wood. It doesn't matter if the carving is coarse and amateurish, because the sentiment is in the personal and thoughtful handmade work. This is the ultimate in an old-fashioned, romantic declaration of love. He can then get this piece of loving wood framed to hang in the bedroom as an etched reminder of the night, and of your everlasting feelings for each other.

Present your gifts to each other in bed, after making love. It's traditional and loving, and all about the two of you.

Flower Power

"The bed should have a canopy above it, with garlands and bunches of flowers. There should be at least two pillows. And a separate couch, perfume, musical instruments, fruits and games."

Kama Sutra

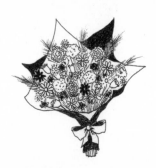

Pleasure Pantry Ingredients

Flowers, flowers and more flowers, of many colors and varieties
Dinner—take out or home-cooked (your choice)
Candles (floral-scented optional)
Music
Oil burner
Essential oil of floral variety of choice (rose and jasmine are good for romance, love and passion)
White bed sheets
Floral-print pillows
Fruity wine
Perfume
Massage oil (floral fragrance of choice)

Preparation

When a woman receives flowers, they make her feel special. Flowers are romantic and thoughtful, and most women would love to receive fresh bouquets of flowers, or even a single hand-picked flower, far more often than they do. Women love getting flowers on special occasions, and they especially love them when they are unexpected, because they are then simply a heart-warming reminder, from the one they love, to say they are thinking of them.

Many men love giving women flowers. They either love flowers themselves, or they love seeing the response flowers can bring to their loved one. To prepare for this special evening, filled with flowers and love, the most important errand to run is to the florist.

Say it to her with flowers:

Red rose	passion
Red tulip	declaration of love
Red poppy	pleasure
Red carnation	admiration
Jonquil	love me
Camellia	perfection
Ivy	eternal fidelity
Forget-me-not	true love, memories
Primrose	I can't live without you
Gladiolus	love at first sight
Stephanotis	happiness in marriage

After getting all the flowers (lots and lots and lots of them), and gathering all the other necessary ingredients for this night of passion, tenderness and caring—including organizing dinner, complete with the meal being set out with flowers on the table, and even on the plates—begin to set the house with the delightful fragrance and stunning visual appeal of flowers in every room. Put a bunch of flowers in every room of your house—even the rooms she won't go into that night, because when she does see them later she'll be reminded of the night you shared. Make sure to put flowers even in the bathroom—no room should be unadorned.

Take flower petals (either purchase separate petals from the florist, or buy bunches specifically for taking all the petals off) and scatter them in a trail from the dining room to the bedroom, leading onto the bed. Also line little candles along the same trail to the base of the bed, so that you can turn off the lights and still see the petals in a romantic aura. Add candles around the bedroom at varying heights and locations: put them on the bedside tables, the dressing table and chest of drawers. Put little tea lights in any potted plants, or on dishes or saucers on the floor.

Choose some romantic music, light the oil burner to create a floral fragrance in the room before she comes home, and set the bed with plain white bed sheets, turned down, and decorated simply with a few floral-print pillows and fresh flower petals. Put plenty of flower petals in the bed and all over the sheets, as you'll be making love on them later. Layer the bed with a variety of soft, colorful, very fragrant petals. Plain white sheets, rather than your regular sheets, are important, because some flowers can release color that will stain sheets. Use sheets that you don't mind staining, and if you use white ones, you can create a color stain of your love-making that, if you ever use the sheets again, will remind you of this night, and this ultra-romantic experience.

Bring to Boil

Arrange, on no particularly special day, for no particular reason, to have a huge bunch of flowers delivered to your lovee. Attach a card with a romantic sentiment of your own, or, if you have trouble with romantic expression, ask the florist for suggestions. Or write, "I have kissed every one of these flowers, so in receiving them you not only have my love and thoughts always of you, but also all the kisses they carry." Don't give any hint of the incredibly romantic night you have planned. For now, let her simply think that your romantic gesture starts and ends with a wonderful surprise bunch of flowers. She'll likely hum and smile all the way home, holding her delightful bunch of flowers, and when she arrives through the front door she'll be in for an even greater romantic surprise.

Lead her into the house and settle her with a nice chilled glass of fruity wine. Present her with dinner, adorned with flowers and petals all over the table and around the plates. If she's blown away and wide-eyed, and notices the candles and petals leading to the bedroom, don't satiate her curiosity, just tell her that she'll discover what comes next a little later. This will build her sense of heightened romance and sexual arousal. Distract her curiosity by giving her a gift, wrapped in a box and decorated with a flower. Let her open the bottle of floral perfume you've chosen for her, and, when she thanks you for it, tell her that you look forward to smelling it on her because you chose it especially to celebrate her on this night—which is no night in particular, just a night when you want to show her how much you love her.

Once you've finished dinner, let her enjoy a little more of the wine, and take this opportunity to go into the bedroom to light all the candles and put the music on. (And on a practical note: this evening is about romance, so leave the dishes and cleaning up for the morning!)

Return to her, take her hand and lead her to the bedroom. Invite her onto the bed and begin to kiss her. Tell her that this night is all about her. Slowly undress her and lay her down against the petal-covered sheet. Take some of the floral-scented massage oil and stroke her from her neck across her shoulders, down her arms, back up and then down her sides, and up her front and around her breasts. Kiss her breasts as you massage them. Rub your hands down past her navel, then skim over her pelvis, very lightly, as a tease and massage her legs down to her feet. Reach your hands under her body, just above her bottom, and rub and reach firmly upwards along her back. Repeat the same movement, starting from underneath her shoulders down to her lower back. Then, using a lighter touch, trace your fingers around her nipples and begin kissing them.

Pick some petals from the bed and lightly shower them across her front. Scatter them lower and lower, while kissing lower and lower, until you reach her mound of Venus. Gently spread her legs and unfurl her lower lips with your fingers while kissing and caressing them. Suck the bud of her clitoris, and lightly flick the velvety soft inner sides of her lips with your tongue. Bring her to a ripe peak, treating every inch of her sexiness as if she were a beautiful flower, and you want to inhale and touch every delicate part. Make love to her against the petals, crushing and smearing them with your rhythmic movements.

Enjoy the fragrance from the crumpled flowers beneath you, released by your motions in the bed. Afterwards, spoon and give her a soft back massage, smelling the floral scent left on her from you making love to her. Tell her how much you love this scent and how you'll remember it always.

Prove to her that nights like this aren't just in fantasies: they're part of real life. Your romantic life together.

Extra Zing

Arrange to have a bouquet of flowers sent to her each day for a week, with each bouquet getting more extravagant every day. Attach cards that start with "I love you because . . ." and list your many different reasons and appreciations, in no particular sequence. Send the last bouquet on Friday, with a card reading, "I love you because it's Friday. And soon we'll have the whole weekend together. And I'll be saved from constantly missing your everything."

Champagne Bubble Bath

Two in the tub for old-style sparkling romance.

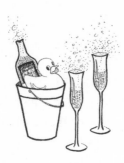

Pleasure Pantry Ingredients

Expensive champagne—1 bottle
Cooler/bottle chiller
Champagne flutes—2
Music/CD player
Candles
Bubble bath (in champagne bottle—optional)
Bath or essential oil of jasmine and/or ylang ylang
Cheap sparkling white wine—2 bottles
Bath pillows—2
Strawberries
Soft washcloths and bath mitts
Shampoo and conditioner (fruit-scented)
Small pail
White terry towelling robes
Towels
Strawberry and champagne Honey Body Dust
Perfume/cologne (optional)
Short side table (optional)

Preparation

Treat yourselves to the luxury of a hot, bubbly bath together. Don't simply regard this bath time as relaxing, but much, much more. Make it an extravagant gesture of old-style glamor and romance: instead of simply sipping champagne in the bath ... have a lavish champagne bubble bath—literally.

If you don't have a bath at home, rent a hotel room or take a weekend away where you can indulge in a bath—even better if you can find a wonderful retreat with a private bath with a view.

You may like to plan and prepare your erotic champagne extravagance together, or surprise your partner on the night. Either way, not much advance preparation is needed, save to gather the ingredients.

Buy your champagne, strawberries and bath accessories, and select your music. If you plan in advance, you can take your time shopping for just the right bath accessories. Many stores have bubble bath gel packaged in mock Champagne bottles, and this is a nice thematic touch if you can find it. Once you have everything, on the night itself adorn the bathroom with candles all around the tub. You may wish to set a small, low table next to the tub and place a variety of candles on it, of all heights, sizes and designs. You can get heart-shaped candles, erotic statuesque couple-in-embrace candles, candles of different scents ... create an artistic, eclectic design of candles next to the tub to conceive a romantic and beautiful atmosphere.

Bring to Boil

Run the bath and, as it's filling, add a whole bottle of bubble bath gel. Don't scrimp—this is a luxurious, extravagant night—splurge! In addition to the bubble bath, you may like to add essential oils of jasmine and ylang ylang. According to aromatherapy principles, jasmine instils a sense of romance when smelled, and ylang ylang has long been associated with increasing sexual desire in men and women.

Stir the bath until the bubbles are nearly pouring over the edge of the tub, and, right before you and your lover get in the bath, take one of the bottles of sparkling wine and pour it in. While one bottle isn't exactly like bathing in an entire tub of champagne, seeing the bubbly splash onto your already frothy bath can add that extra bit of indulgence and really set the mood for pleasure and excess.

Step into the bath together and start soaking it in.

You and your lovee can lean against each other or, if you have a big tub, you can each lean against your bath pillows and truly relax. Pop the expensive bottle of champagne and pour each other a glass. Feed each other strawberries. Fluff bubbles onto each other's skin and wet each other with the hot, slippery, bubbly, scented water. Kiss. Perfect the art of kissing together—research has shown that lovers consider kissing to be one of the most essential aspects of an intimate relationship, yet they conversely report that there is not enough kissing in their relationship. Women, in particular, stated that the pleasure they receive from kissing is close to the best pleasure they get from any kind of sexual expression or activity. But it's certainly not just women hankering for more luscious lip-locking: a survey of 4000 men revealed that kissing was their favorite part of foreplay, and most men want more kissing with their lover.

Time in a sexy bath together is one of the most ideal settings to treat yourselves to a lover-ly kissing session. Give each other teasing kisses, wet kisses and body-sliding kisses. Have a conversation with your lips, giving each other short and long kisses and counter-kisses. Kiss your lover's neck, forehead, eyelids, cheeks, ears, hair, throat and chest. Suck their nipples and play with their bodies under the warm, bubbly water. Pour the second bottle of sparkling wine into the bath for a top-up of bubbly and sexy champers aroma.

When you're ready, take the shampoo and wash each other's hair. Slowly lather their hair, taking at least five minutes each to give the other a scrumptious scalp massage as you work the lather in. Take the small bath pail and pour water slowly over their head to wash the shampoo off. Then work the conditioner into their scalp and let it soak in while you use some extra conditioner in your hands to reach down and rub some of the slippery smoothness into their lower love zones. He can tickle her clit with come-hither motions and rub up and down, as well as making firm circles all around her mons, lips, clitoral hood and glans. She can use the slickness of the water-and-conditioner combination to her skilful advantage, using both hands to weave and rub liberally up and down his shaft as he gets harder and harder in response.

As the bubbles in the bath start disappearing, and the bubbling anticipation of more full-body caressing takes over, step out of the bath and into your luxurious white terry towelling robes. The robes are optional (unless you already own them), but wrapping yourselves into fluffy white robes can bring a connotation of vacations, relaxation and spoiling each other, plus it's a nice transition from an extravagant bath to your bedroom.

Towel each other off, and as you cross to the bedroom, bring some of the candles with you to maintain the loving light to bask in as you make love.

When you're dry, cap off the opulence of the night by lightly dusting each other's bodies with some of the strawberry and champagne-flavored Honey Body Dust. The Honey Body Dust is available from many sex shops as well as select body, beauty and lingerie shops. Sprinkle the bed sheets with the "scentual" dust and, using your fingers or a feather, brush the sensual dust all over each other, leaving a silky-soft glow on each other's skin.

Continue your kissing conversation, more intensely now, and make love side by side facing each other, or in the spooning position, so both of you get ample opportunity to enjoy the scent of the bath, the champagne and the Honey Dust, on each other. Drink each other in and enjoy.

Extra Zing

Buy a new bottle of perfume or cologne for your lovee. Choose a fragrance they have never worn before. Give it to them, gift-wrapped in a box and bow, in the bath, to really spoil them. Spritz it on them after they are dry, and make love while they are wearing this new scent. It will create a wonderful, loving memory, easily remembered by you both, because the sense of smell is a powerful trigger for memories. Each time they wear this new gift it will evoke the experience of this night, of the unique, sensual, sumptuous experience shared between you, between bubbles and between the sheets.

Score!

Yes, yes, yes!

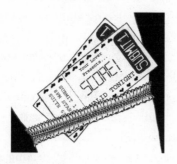

Pleasure Pantry Ingredients

Sporting event tickets
Sporting team paraphernalia:
  Sport or team jumpers/jerseys
  Sport or team scarf
  Knee-high socks of team colors
  Mascot trinkets
  Sport or team beer can-holders

G-string and bra in team/sport colors
Hairspray paint in team/sport colors
Hotel reservations (hotel requirement: cable TV with international sports channels and broadcasts)

Preparation

Even without flowers and chocolates in sight, romance can be just as sweet, and sweeter even, if measured by pure thoughtfulness. One of the reasons women often don't romance men—along with the ancient gender stereotype some people cling to that says it's the man's role to woo, court and romance—is that women are pretty sure that their man isn't going to like the traditional romantic scene, or that it wouldn't be his number one choice of a way to spend more than a few hours.

Not so with sport. Men love their sports (a vast majority of them, anyway). They are lovingly faithful to their teams over an entire lifetime, from childhood to old age. They are fiercely devoted to never missing a game or match, to remembering history, significant dates, amazing experiences and memorable moments. They are passionate about sports —very, *very* passionate. Combine you, your man, sports and all that passion, and as sure as a race's starter gun exploding, you've got a recipe for hot romance.

Prepare to knock his socks off by making all the arrangements for the day and night, and then surprising him with them. When a good home game is scheduled for his favorite team, make arrangements for great seats. Get all the team gear from jerseys to scarves, socks, banners, flags and mascot trinkets. Buy a new G-string and bra set in the team colors. Also buy some colored hairspray in the team colors and, just for fun, secretly spray your pubic hair in stripes of each of the team colors the morning of the big game.

Adjust your ingredients to suit your man's favorite sport. If it's not football, soccer or some similar team sport, you can still have fun creating a teasing sexy theme while taking him to tennis, motocross, speedboat racing, wrestling, hockey, golf, and so on.

Bring to Boil

On the morning of the big event, surprise him with breakfast in bed and attach the match tickets to the front page of the sports section of the morning paper. When he finds them, tell him that you've got the whole day planned, and it's all a surprise; all he has to do is get dressed. As he's showering, pack an overnight bag for the two of you with the bare essentials needed before you get back home tomorrow, including your new team-themed G-string and bra. Throw the bag in the trunk of your car, or, if you're not driving, even more reason to pack a minimal amount as you'll be carrying it all day until you get to the hotel. Lay out all the team gear on the bed so he knows that both of you are totally embracing the theme of the day and showing your team support, as well as just having some good, clean fun wearing his favorite team colors together.

Before you get to the match, place some sexual bets on the outcome of the game. You might each bet on what the final score is, and what the quarter- and half-time scores are, or how much you think your team will win by. Bet sexual acts you want your lover to do to you should you win.

At the match, throw diets aside and indulge in all the traditional sporting event food. Never mind "proper nutrition" today: chow down on the hotdogs, peanuts, nachos and chips. Drink beer in plastic cups. Romance doesn't have to mean glamor and refinement—sometimes the simple things in life are the best. And today it's sports and sausages, fun and french fries, and beer and bonding.

When the game is over, and you've cheerily enjoyed every minute of it, take charge and lead your man to the hotel room you've booked. Check in, open a few beers from the minibar, and put them in the team-themed can holders from your bag. Celebrate if your team won, but if they didn't, tell him that he's the winner tonight, because he's in for more surprises.

Leave him sitting on the bed in anticipation, with the remote to the TV, so he can plug in to even more sport from around the world. In the bathroom, change into your G-string and bra, add the team-colored jersey on top, and put on the team's striped knee-high socks. (If you can't get the socks, a spicy substitution is a pair of garters peeking out from below the team jersey.) Emerge from the bathroom with a flirty smirk and, when you have his attention, ask, "Ready to play?"

Go over to him and straddle his lap to distract him from the TV. Leave the sport on the TV on as a thematic touch in the background and push him onto the bed. Strip him down and take off your jersey, but for a while pleasure him wearing just your lingerie and team knee-high socks. When he's about ready to scream—in frustration rather than victory—slip your panties off, show him your color-themed hair with a laugh, and then ride him until he pops his "gland finale." Yes! Score!

Order room service, watch sports on TV together and place more "double or nothing" sexual bets. Round two: winner cashes in on the sexual bets. *Ding ding ding!*

Extra Zing
For an added thrill to your sporting good time as a romantic couple, take a risk and feel the rush of adrenaline together by taking up an extreme sport as a couple. Consider skydiving, scuba diving, snowboarding, rock climbing, rodeo lessons, racing car driving school, or even tandem bungee jumping. If this is too extreme for you, join a mixed club sporting team together. It is great exercise and a fun way to bond in a common hobby, plus exercise is critical for healthy sexual function. Men and women both need good muscle tone throughout their lives for good physiological arousal and

orgasm, as well as a healthy circulatory system for good blood flow to the genitals to maintain a long life of solid sexual function.

You could, as a couple, agree to run a marathon or fun run together, and train several times a week, for months in advance, working together towards a common goal. Coach each other on: "Come on!" "Do it!" "Harder!" and "Faster!" may mean something slightly different in this context, but the training is good for you, and the time spent together is even better. Life is an adventure: live it together.

L'amour

Ooh la la . . . ooh love, love, love

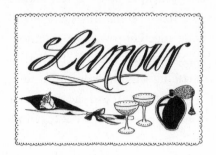

Pleasure Pantry Ingredients

French cuisine
French couture lingerie
French perfume
French men's cologne
French films
Candles
Beautiful gift card and gift boxes
A single red rose
French champagne
French white wine
Book of French poetry (optional)
Tickets to Paris (optional)

Preparation

The French are among the world's most prolific lovers, having sex quite a bit more often than many others. Americans have sex between 70 and 112 times per year on average, while the French notch up 137 times per year.

This night of l'*amour* isn't about how often you make love, though: it's a night of French-themed classic romance. The fanciful excitement of the eve is through the idea and reality of your romantic love for each other, not the stereotypical fantasy of the "French maid costume." In fact, less than 10 percent of the French dress up in the bedroom so, to be truly authentic French lovers for the night, stick with the classics.

To prepare a special night for her, shop for just the right, and very special, ingredients. If you are not a master at cooking French food, make dinner reservations at a romantic French restaurant. Buy a new set of couture or high-end French lingerie as a special surprise for your lover. Make sure you get the right size by taking a set of lingerie she already owns into the shop with you. Different brands of lingerie can have slightly different sizing, so it's best if you have a sample size from which to select your new foxy French outfit of choice for her. Choose something you know she'll feel beautiful in, as well as something you want to see her in (and take off her). To get the absolute best French lingerie, choose something from:

Chantal Thomass

Les Folies d'Elodie

La Perla—French couture-inspired range

Agent Provocateur—'Frenchy' line

Dior

Also buy French fragrances, choosing one for her and one for you with this romantic evening and theme in mind. Classic and popular French perfumes for you to select from are:

Chanel No 5

J'adore by Christian Dior

Love in Paris by Nina Ricci

Mure & Musc by Annick Goutal
Rive Gauche by Yves Saint Laurent
Ambre Sultan by Serge Lutens

And for a scent for you:

Pour un Homme by Caron
Patchouli by Guerlain
Eau Sauvage by Christian Dior

Rent a few French films, choosing from titles such as:

Belle de Jour
Mon Homme
La Piscine
Le Zèbre
37.2° le Matin
Trois Couleurs: Bleu
Trois Couleurs: Rouge
Trois Couleurs: Blanc

Also make sure you have plenty of candles placed around the bedroom. If you look carefully through specialty candle shops, you may find candles decorated with images of Moulin Rouge dancing girls, and old-fashioned 1920s and '30s pictures of women strolling down the street holding parasols, as in the film *Gigi*, or even mini prints of classic French impressionist paintings.

Put a book of French poetry on the bedside table, and practice reading a few in your best and most suave French accent (without being ridiculous). Wrap your gifts of perfume and lingerie in beautiful boxes, with a card that says, "*Je t'aime*. From your adoring *minou*." (*Minou* means "kitten" and is a loving, flirtatious pet name French women call their sweet, romantic man. Own this affectionate pet name and let her call you it all night if she wants.) Leave the card and presents on the bed for her to discover and unwrap when she gets home.

As a final touch, do as the romantic French men do and select a stunning single red rose to present to your love.

Bring to Boil

When your lover arrives home from work, surprise her at the door—or train station or bus stop—with the red rose. Take her into your arms and give her a French kiss, starting lightly at first before becoming persistent and desirous with your tongue. No pecks here—tonight is about demonstratively expressing your passion and love. Even if you don't speak French, the language of love is understood by all lovers. Welcome her home, calling her *ma beauté* (my beauty), *mon trésor* (my treasure), *mon ange* (my angel), or the classic French lover's pet name, *chérie* (darling). Shower her with kisses and murmurings of sweet love in French. Ask her to put on something sexy and beautiful, because you're taking her out for a romantic dinner.

Lead her into the bedroom, and let her see the exquisite designer boxes waiting for her to open. Encourage her to open them right then and there, and insist she wear their contents tonight, as you bought them especially for the occasion—the occasion being nothing in particular, except to spoil and adore her. Ask her to give you a teasing peek at her in the new lingerie, so all evening you can envision how seductively she's dressed from the inside out. Appreciate the lingerie on her with lots of flattering declarations of "*Très belle! Très jolie! Ooh la la!*" and kiss her hand to your lips as if she's too delectable to resist, then walk away saying that if you stay and watch her dress, she'll never get dressed.

Head out to the restaurant. Order a bottle of Veuve Clicquot to share, and then confidently and charmingly order the meal for both of you. For traditional and authentic romantic French fare, start your meal with *foie gras truffe* and *toast chaud*, followed by *plateau de fruits de mer* (seafood platter). A truly French seafood platter will have *huitres* (oysters), *oursins* (sea urchin), clams and *homard* (lobster). Then order the *plateau de fromages* (including *chèvre*, Camembert and Roquefort) before ending with a light dessert. Choose from such lip-smacking options as *tartelettes aux fraises, duo de mousse chocolate blanc chocolate noir*, or *soufflé au* Grand Marnier.

Once you have finished dining as if you were in France itself, continue your sensual experience of all things French back at home. Once there, you can ask her to open a bottle of French white wine of choice from the fridge, while you light the candles in the bedroom. Sip the wine and enjoy watching her undress down to her couture lingerie. Make love by starting with, of course, *soixante-neuf* (69), before moving on to making love *en cuillere*, which is the spooning position, with her in front nestled against him as he penetrates from behind her. Curl into each other, before finishing in the *classique* French position *la levrette*, which is man-on-top, lying against her with complete body contact. French kiss throughout your lovemaking, and afterwards also.

When completely satiated, lie back and enjoy a final glass of wine. As you both sip the wine, you can reach over to the bedside table and take the book of French poetry, romancing her even more by reading a few poems to her. It doesn't matter if you don't speak French; just enjoy the sounds of the words and the romance of the French language. Or else, simply read one romantic French poem by 1930s French poet Paul Eluard:

J'ai regardé devant moi
Dans la foule je t'ai vue
Parmi les blés je t'ai vue
Sous un arbre je t'ai vue

Au bout de tous mes voyages
Au fond de tous mes tourments
Au tournant de tous les rires
Sortant de l'eau et du feu

L'été, l'hiver je t'ai vue
Dans ma maison je t'ai vue
Entre mes bras je t'ai vue
Dans mes rêves, je t'ai vue

Je ne te quitterai plus.

Translation:

I looked ahead
In the crowd I saw you
In the corn field I saw you
Under a tree I saw you

At the end of all my journeys
At the bottom of all my torments
Around the corner of laughter
Emerging from the water and the fire

In summer, in winter I saw you
In my house I saw you
In my arms I saw you
In my dreams I saw you

I will never leave you.

And when she's totally swept off her feet, lie back and relax together, capping off the night by enjoying a French dramatic or erotic film in bed. Ah, *bon.*

Extra Zing

Dream about going to France together—or make it a reality and surprise your lovee with tickets to Paris. Stroll the Parisian streets taking in the music, wine, food, art, fashion and ambience. Rent a villa in the south of France for a few weeks to live out the fantasy of an ultimate romantic getaway. If a trip to Paris, the city of love, isn't possible for a while, surprise her with the essence of French love and arrange to have a signature perfume sent from the uniquely luxurious perfumery L'Artisan Parfumeur. There are international retailers outside France or, if one isn't near you, shop at their online boutique. As an extra-special gift, you can give her a voucher for the two of you to attend one of their famous perfume workshops, to design a fragrance that is uniquely reflective of your love. Either way, a gift from L'Artisan Parfumeur is to be cherished, and she'll love having a treasure of Paris sitting on her dresser, and whenever she wears the perfume, she'll know you chose it especially for her, and especially to remind her of your French desires and dreams.

Cosmic Union

Sacred, sensual, spiritual sex

Pleasure Pantry Ingredients
Flowing, colorful pieces of fabric
Pillows of varying shapes, sizes and colors
Flowers
Vases
Incense/oil burner
Candles
Music
Tantric workshop (optional)

Preparation
To experience an enhanced level of lovemaking, introduce each other to the world of Tantric sex. Tantra in the modern Western world has come to mean experiencing a spiritual connection with sexuality; however, Tantra is much more than that. Originally it came from Hindu and Buddhist practices aimed at achieving enlightenment, and sexual practice was one of those paths. Tantra literally means "weaving" or "expanding," and Tantric practitioners will describe how they feel interwoven with their partner, and how their pleasure expands through their bodies, and between them

and their lover, and then upwards to a spiritual harmony well beyond the physical sensations felt during lovemaking.

To prepare, first create a sacred space for love. Adorn your bedroom with flowing fabrics on the floor, walls, bed head and over the bed. Place an assortment of at least ten pillows on the bed so that it feels luxurious and inviting. Take lots of flowers and scatter them around the room—loose and in vases. Use incense or an oil burner to create a beautiful aroma in the room. Light candles all around the room, perhaps in a circle around the bed, to create a temple effect in which you worship each other and your love.

Make sure you and your lovee have several hours alone with no distractions. Tantric sex can be lovingly enjoyed in the morning, day or night—the right time to do it is simply when you choose to let go and share together.

Bring to Boil

The Tantric approach to lovemaking entails stimulating your energy before relaxing into tranquil, slow lovemaking. One of the best ways to stimulate your sexual energy together is through dancing. Tantric sex principles say that fast dancing is best for drawing up and releasing energy, so choose some music you can really move to. Once you feel charged up together you can scale down to softer music for a little bit of slow dancing. Enjoy the feeling of being pressed up against each other as you dance, and cheek to cheek, chest to chest, focus on your breathing and each other's breath. Sway together until you start to notice a mutual breathing rhythm. This starts the connecting process between you, mingling your breath and body movements in tandem.

The next stage is to slow down your bodies even more while still maintaining a high focus on cultivating sexual energy in each other's bodies. Tantric practices to do this generally focus on awakening the seven chakras in the body.

The chakras are described by Tantric practitioners as wheels of energy that represent various aspects of ourselves. There is a vast and complex network of energy centres in the body which filter into the seven main points, and most Tantric sex practice involves concentrating on and stimulating those seven centres to bring about total mind-body-spirit awareness and pleasure.

To give loving attention to your chakras, both of you lie down naked on the bed of pillows. If the air is cold, cover yourselves with a cosy blanket or one of the light, sensual fabrics. Taking turns, give your lovee sensual touch all over using feathery fingertip movements to stimulate them all over their skin. Move from the base chakra upwards (see the following table for details), not with the purpose of physical sexual pleasure at this point but purely the sensation of touch, without response or immediate reciprocation. As the receiver, you can enhance your mind-body-spirit awareness by visualizing the associated chakra colors as you are caressed by your lover.

The Chakra System

Chakra	Color	Meditation
Root (base of spine)	red	balance and grounding
Sexual (genitals)	orange	passion
Solar plexus	yellow	your dynamic sense of self
Heart	green	love and compassion
Throat	blue	creativity and inner truth

| Brow (third eye) | violet | wisdom |
| Crown (top of head) | white | connection with divine love |

As you give and receive loving touch, imagining the colors around you and meditating on the associations with the energy centers, breathe in and out deeply. In Tantra, the breath is the key to channelling energy throughout the body.

From sensual body touching, the next movement together is exchanging loving gazes, before worshipping each other through kissing. Sit across from each other and look lovingly into each other's eyes. With your hot breath, blow on your partner's shoulders and neck, then embrace in a melting kiss. The process and philosophy of Tantra is to connect, rather than race headlong into intercourse and orgasm, so spend quite a bit of time together simply leaning into each other and connecting your whole upper bodies. Wrap your arms around each other and feel your hearts beating together.

The art of Tantric lovemaking requires you to connect from bottom to top, not just through genital contact. You may wish to make love lying down (in any position), with full-body contact from tip to toe, or sitting propped up by pillows. Feel the initial pleasure through mutual genital massage and penetration, slowly rocking your pelvises in a pleasurable rhythm for you both. Meditate on the sensations of pleasure radiating upwards through your bodies, from your lower chakras through to those in the head. When you feel warmth reach your heart chakra, press each other's hands against your hearts to bring full awareness that your lovemaking has transcended physical genital touch, and you're opening your hearts fully to each other, present in the moment. Maintain your physical stimulation while gazing into each other's eyes.

While Tantric sex doesn't attach itself to any goal, many Tantric practitioners like to communicate with their lover so that when they do want to experience orgasm, they come together as a couple, united wholly and soul-ly. Ask your lover if they're ready to peak with you, and then stimulate her yoni pearl (clitoris), and rub and rock against his lingam (penis) until you both ride the wave of bliss together. Lie together in a state of deep relaxation, enjoying the lingering touch and connection with each other. Treasure the gift of your shared love and union.

Extra Zing

Sign yourselves up for a weekend Tantric workshop. There are many teachers to choose from, and most offer intensive weekend workshops for couples to open their hearts to divine love for each other, and to learn the art of Tantric love-making. Some couples who are curious about Tantric sex and want to learn more—especially with a teacher there on hand to guide them through the exercises—worry that a work-shop will be too intense, or too nude. Most Tantric work-shops, especially for beginners, are never conducted in the nude. All exercises are taught fully clothed, and many cou-ples report feeling as connected after just two days at the workshop as they were when they first fell in love. Even more so sometimes, because they discover a whole new cosmic dimension to their feelings for each other, and a spir-itual bond they share not just inside the bedroom, but in life.

The Perfumed Garden

Plant a delightful garden bed of love together.

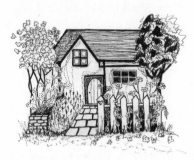

Pleasure Pantry Ingredients

Seedlings of:
  Basil
  Lavender
  Gardenia
  Geranium
  Rose

Cutting of a frangipani tree
Gardening boots—2 pairs
Overalls (for him)
Gardener's tool belt
Gardener's apron
Gardening gloves—2 pairs
Spade
Wood saw
Nails
Hammer
Fertilizer
Wooden boards for garden-bed edging
Paint (orange, pink, red, white and/or purple)
Paintbrushes
Stencil patterns (optional)
Picnic hamper
Picnic blanket

Preparation

Along with the Kama Sutra and the Ananga Ranga, *The Perfumed Garden* is one of the world's most famous erotic books. Written by Sheikh Nefzawi during the fifteenth century in Tunis, it has long been regarded as a poetic, erotic, richly detailed and entertaining sensual guide for lovers. Its aim was to stimulate and maintain passion for all men and women, by describing variations of male and female erotic bodies as well as effective arousal techniques and positions. Later translated by Sir Richard Burton, *The Perfumed Garden* has become a classic in the erotica genre.

Create your own perfumed garden of love together. Pick a sunny, gorgeous weekend day in spring and spend it outside together. If you live in an apartment, build a mini garden box for your windowsill and spend the day at nurseries gathering your seedlings, then afterwards head to a park for a picnic to continue your romantic day in a garden setting. Choose all or some of the plants from the ingredients list—according to research, each of them have love-enhancing and libido-stimulating effects. Once you have gathered your gardening materials and picnic, wander down into your garden, where delights await you . . .

Bring to Boil

You're going to work up a sweat, so wear correct gardening gear—but with a sexy twist. He can wear overalls without a shirt, to show off his torso, and strap on a gardening belt— it doesn't matter what kind, as women love a man in a tool belt! She can also go topless, covering herself with a gardening apron complete with a tool set of her own.

Choose the location for your garden bed and measure it out. One of you can start building the wooden edging, sawing and nailing the pieces together, while the other digs the ground to turn the soil over and then adds the fertilizer. You want your garden bed to be fertile, for your sexy, beautiful flowers to grow well together. Once the edging is done, you can paint it with colors that will coordinate with the blossoms you're planting, such as white, pink, red, orange and purple. You can leave your edging with a solid color or two, or, if you really want to be romantic, get a little creative and artistic with the love garden that you're planting together: draw stripes, swirls and a trail of love hearts of differing sizes and pairings along the edging, perhaps a couple with your initials in them. If you're not confident in your artistic abilities, you can use a stencil pattern bought at a store. Then, in one discreet corner, write the date and each sign it under "Planted with love."

Add your seedlings in a joint effort, planting them with your hands together, pressing into the soil, and spacing the seedlings out in a pattern that will allow each plant to grow well. You may like to start with your basil plant. Perhaps it seems unusual to add basil to your love garden of beautiful flowers, but basil is actually one of the key herbs of love, from its leaves to its flowers. In the Middle Ages, a legend was born that associated basil with faithful love. The story goes that a young girl died and left behind her adoring and desperate lover, who cried over her grave every day. He shed countless tears, and one day a basil flower began to grow from his tears. His tears wet the flower bud every day until it blossomed, and a lovely, sweet, delicate perfume wafted from it, which he enjoyed and felt it reminiscent of her.

From that legend, other stories grew around the sensual and loving properties of the sweet smell of the basil flower. Basil then became a central ingredient in many love spells and erotic rituals. One ritualized the rubbing of shredded and powdered basil flowers on one's lover's chest to ensure that they were always faithful and loving. Over time, Arabs and Europeans alike used basil to awaken the passions in their lover. Even Sheikh Nefzawi, in *The Perfumed Garden*, wrote of the sensual benefits of using basil massage oil, comparing this delicate herb with a woman's body, explaining that "both have to be first stirred with the nails, to reach a high state of pleasure." Once you have planted your basil seedling, you may like to echo the sentiment of the basil-faithful-loving ritual by plucking a tiny leaf, tearing it in two and each rubbing the essence of your half on your lovee's chest. Seal your ritual with a kiss.

Plant your lavender seedling next. Lavender has been shown to increase lust in both men and women—especially in men. In fact, tests have shown that the aroma of lavender is not only relaxing but invigorating to the sexual response, creating a measurable physiological response of increased blood flow to the genitals, and increased lust and libido. Plant the lavender so that, when it blossoms, you can add sprigs of it to a little vase in your bedroom, knowing not only its effect but that you planted it together.

Finally, adorn your garden bed of love with colorful flowers. The gardenia and frangipani have fragrances that elicit an aphrodisiac response in lovers; these flowers have long been associated with sweet-smelling love. Geraniums are associated with warming a heart, and long-lasting love. Roses, the most famous romantic flower throughout time

and literature, can be planted as a reflection of, and investment in, your own growing love.

> *Lovers now send a single silken rose, perfumed*
> *and sealed into a plastic shell.*
> *Is love so desperate to fend off change?*
> *Better a rose still wet with rain, smelling of*
> *summer and ephemeral. Speaking of living*
> *love. Speaking of other summers yet to come.*
> (Pam Brown)

Invest in each other. Invest in your future together, and more
seasons to be enjoyed and shared together. Plant your rose
seedlings, and then give each other a kiss. Make love right
there in the setting of your love garden, or at home, under
your flower-box windowsill, if you live in an apartment.
Spread your picnic blanket out in front of your newly
planted garden bed and make love, as they did in *The Perfumed
Garden*. Try the "frog position," as outlined in this erotic sex
manual. He sits while she lies on her back with her pelvis in
his lap, draping her legs over his shoulders (or around his
shoulders or waist). He grinds his pelvis and, holding her
hips, can guide her rhythm up and down him as well. To
help bring her to climax, he can also reach straight down
and work her clitoris until she arches and opens her hips
wide and climaxes in his lap. Now flushed and radiant, relax
and enjoy your romantic picnic together, lying naked with
your gardening tools around you and your garden bed of
love as your backdrop. Plant the memory of this day together
as one you'll remember each time you enjoy your growing
garden, and your thriving love.

Extra Zing

For an added investment and loving touch to your garden of love, plant a "love capsule." Build, or buy, a small box and in it place mementos of your past year together. Include ticket stubs, a few photographs, wrapping from treasured presents and love notes to each other about what the year together has meant to you. Read them to each other before placing them in the box.

Seal the box and bury it in the back of your love garden bed before planting your seedlings in front of it. If you're an urban couple planting a small windowsill box, make a miniature version of the love capsule.

Promise to make this day your love anniversary, and on this day each year dig up your love capsule, go through your love treasures, cherishing the memories with each other, and then add another year of your mementos before returning the capsule back to your garden of love.

Chocolate Obsession

Sweet, velvety, irresistible . . . you melt in my mouth.

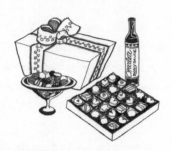

Pleasure Pantry Ingredients

Chocolate treats—you and your lover's favorites to nibble on
Hershey's Chocolate Kisses
Thick chocolate body frosting
Chocolate sauce
Chocolate liqueur/crème de cacao
Chocolate marshmallow body butter
Chocolate and strawberry edible underwear set
Chocolate nipple drops
Chocolate body dust
Chocolate body paint
Hot chocolate for two
Candles
Red bed sheet

Preparation

Why we love chocolate:

"Chocolate makes otherwise normal people melt into strange
states of ecstasy." (John West)

"Chocolate is heavenly, mellow, sensual, deep. Dark, sumptuous, gratifying, potent, dense, creamy, seductive, suggestive,
rich, excessive, silky, smooth, luxurious, celestial. Chocolate is
downfall, happiness, pleasure, love, ecstasy, fantasy. Chocolate
makes us wicked, guilty, sinful, healthy, chic, happy." (Elaine
Sherman)

"Chocolate, of course, is the stuff of which fantasies are made.
Rich, dark, velvety-smooth fantasies that envelop the senses
and stir the passions. Chocolate is madness; chocolate is
delight." (Judith Olney)

"It [chocolate] flatters you for awhile; it warms you for an
instant; then, all of a sudden, it kindles a mortal fever in you."
(Madame de Sevigne, 1620–1705, French courtesan
and writer)

The association between chocolate and romance is ancient.
When chocolate first became popular in Europe many cen-
turies ago, it was believed to invigorate men and make
women less inhibited, immediately rendering it a popular
gift between sweethearts to heat up any possible blossoming
romance. The cacao (or cocoa) bean comes from the cacao
tree, which has been cultivated in South America for over
3000 years, and from the outset, whether eaten in food or
boiled into a drink, cacao quickly became known for its
energetic mood-enhancing and stamina-building qualities.
Aztec emperor Montezuma, who lived from 1480–1520,
declared of chocolate: "The divine drink, which builds up
resistance and fights fatigue. A cup of this precious drink
permits a man to walk for a whole day without food."

Modern science has revealed even more information about the particularly sexy qualities of chocolate. In fact, it has two interesting properties that make it an ideal sex enhancer. First, it contains phenylalanine, which is an amino acid that affects arousal and enhances our mood. Dark chocolate in particular can be a vasodilator, meaning it increases blood flow, enhancing not only mood but physical arousal too. Chocolate also contains a chemical called theobromine, which boosts endorphin production. Endorphins target opiate receptors on cell membranes, thereby inducing a sense of pleasure, sometimes extreme and intense pleasure. Chocolate, as it is digested in the body, gives one a feeling of being "high," much like we feel when we are falling in love or tumbling into lust. If chocolate is the food of love, then indulge and play on . . .

To prepare, make sure you've organized your ingredients, notes and deliveries. The more prepared you are in all the details, the sweeter the seduction will be.

Bring to Boil

Because men traditionally court women with romantic gifts of chocolate, switch gears and "flip the script"—take this opportunity to entice him with the sweet seduction of chocolate. After you have gathered all your chocolate ingredients, tempt your lovee all day by sending him tantalizing treats with flirty notes, so he knows there's a sweet surprise in store later that night.

Start in the morning by arranging for a morning mocha coffee to be delivered to his work, with a note from you saying, "A sweet morning mocha for my sweetheart. Drink up and save your energy levels. You'll need them tonight!"

This will immediately start your lover thinking about what may be happening tonight, and smiling because it may seem like a long day's work away yet, but he already can't wait.

If he takes a packed lunch, make sure you put some Chocolate Kisses in it, and also a small tube of thick chocolate body frosting. He'll start to get hot with the hint by now. If your man goes out for lunch, arrange to have the Kisses and body frosting (perhaps wrapped in plain brown wrapping paper, or else love-heart paper) waiting for him on his desk or at his workspace, with another lustful note, when he gets back from lunch. You may have to enlist a coworker or administrative assistant to help with this.

In the afternoon, or before he comes home from work, have a card delivered to his office, attached to one gorgeous piece of gourmet chocolate. On the card, write a sweet love note using your own words, and end it with, "Before you get home for some sweet loving, make sure you bring a few ingredients with you. One: chocolate liqueur or crème de cacao. Two: a bottle of chocolate sauce. See you soon. Taste you soon. xoxo."

Before your lovee gets home, rub some chocolate marshmallow body butter behind your ears and anywhere that it may smell good on your skin—but not in too many places, because you want to save your skin for the eating and licking of the edible chocolate. Also make sure that the bedroom, or lounge—wherever you prefer to play (in winter, a lounge room in front of a fire is a nice place to undress and then wind and unwind together)—is ready with candles lit, red bed sheet laid out (things will get messy, so it's best to buy a simple red sheet, with the knowledge that it may never be used again, and choose a red sheet because it's a color that goes well with the chocolate theme and is sexier than a plain white or floral sheet) and chocolate ingredients seductively displayed.

He probably thought he was coming home with the sole ingredients for the evening's play, so he'll be wildly surprised when he sees that the store-bought chocolate sauce was a ruse, and that you have a plethora of sex-themed chocolate indulgences so you can get hot and sticky together. Tonight, break the rules and have dessert before dinner. Bear in mind one rule, though: the art of making love with chocolate is "less is more." It's easy to get sick from too much chocolate sweetness (yes, really), so go slowly and use hints of chocolate rather than gorging on it.

Lead him into the bedroom or lounge room and unveil your new outfit to him: your tempting "eat-me-please" strawberry and chocolate edible undie and bra set. Before letting him touch and lick, though, lie down together and start your kissing chocolate adoration of each other with a few thick chocolate nipple drops dribbled on you for him to suck off, and a bit of the chocolate frosting and sauce dribbled on you both. Sprinkle some chocolate body dust all over his body as you undress him, and then take the chocolate body paint and decorate his dick and balls before sucking every bit of it off, as if you have an unstoppable chocolate obsession.

After he has come, continue to kiss flirtatiously with chocolate on your lips, and then wiggle and stretch your breasts, in your strawberry and chocolate bra, near his face, and tell him that if he wants to taste your sweetness, tonight it has a chocolate coating which needs licking off before he can dip inside further. Mmmm, yum.

Once you've eaten each other for dessert, you may like to then take a dinner break. Stay messy and sticky and just raid the fridge. Eat on the floor. Go back to your chocolate-stained red sheet and enjoy a postcoital cocktail of crème de cacao, or share a mug of steaming hot chocolate. Be wild, unstructured and spontaneous—as if nothing in this world matters except for the two of you, and mounds and mounds of sex and chocolate.

Extra Zing

Add an extra layer of romantic sweetness by personalizing your relationship in chocolate. Hire a professional choco-latier to custom-make some chocolates for you and your lovee. You may like to order some love-heart chocolates and have them specially decorated with both your initials, or you may like to have a custom mold made. Most designer choco-latiers offer custom-made molds and they can do just about anything from outlines of your portraits, 3D designs of your weddings rings, chocolate flowers, a bed with hearts on it, and even genitalia images if you want to go there.

If there isn't a boutique chocolatier near you, online ordering of any request takes about two weeks. Search the internet for a chocolatier who can do what you want, and between chocolate and your lovee as your muse, design your thoughtful expression of sweet romance for your love.

The Invitation

A lover's tryst

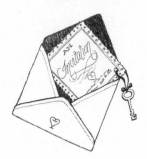

Pleasure Pantry Ingredients
Beautiful invitations—3
Coordinating or matching stationery
Hotel reservations
Flowers
Box of chocolates
Candles—2
New sexy shoulder bag
Lingerie, boxed and wrapped
Wine and cheese
Picture postcard of the hotel, framed
Picture postcard of a romantic destination of choice (optional)

Preparation

Indulge in a weekend of extra-special romance by planning a surprise treat for your lady lovee. Choose a hotel or romantic getaway, and a couple of weeks before the weekend you've chosen to whisk her away, buy your ingredients (except the flowers). Make a special effort to go to a boutique invitation shop to hand-select stunning, intricate, delicate invitations for her: the invitation sets the tone of the weekend.

When you make your hotel reservations, ask to speak to the concierge and explain to them that you have a romantic weekend planned, filled with surprises for your partner, and that you'd like to enlist their help to make sure all the surprises occur without a hitch. Ask if you can email your needs to them so they have them in writing, and everything is clear. Swear them to secrecy!

Treat the weekend away as a romantic fantasy, one in which you are both hot and hungry lovers, almost as if you were engaging in an affair—a hot, loving affair without any guilt. Invite her on the weekend in this teasing way, pretending that you're inviting her to have an affair with you. Injecting your relationship with the essence of an illicit affair can be powerfully alluring, and take you right back to when you first met and couldn't concentrate on anything else but each other; when you were discovering each other, when you had to have each other all the time, as much as possible; when every minute together was exciting. Flirting in this way sends natural amphetamines and endorphins surging through the body. Pack this flirty thrill into your weekend, and experience a hot romance that will spicily invigorate your romantic relationship for weeks and months to come.

Bring to Boil
Here are all the steps for your romantic week.

Monday
Arrange for a bouquet of flowers to be sent to her during the day. Instead of attaching a card, attach your beautiful invitation. In your own handwriting, address it to her first name with her middle name in parentheses. Write, "Please join me

this weekend . . . for an affair to remember. No need to RSVP, simply keep this invitation with you. Wait for further details later in the week. Love . . ." and sign it with your first name, and your middle name (or another name—perhaps a pet name—if you don't have a middle name) in parentheses. She's going to be curious about why you're using both of your first and middle names, but the reason will become clear the next day. You're building the sense of slightly switching identities, to create the effect of having an affair without it being too much of an unrealistic fantasy, because you're still using your own names, just your secondary ones. If she comes home that night and pumps you for more information, simply say, "Didn't the invitation say to await further details later in the week?" and leave it at that. Do not be tempted to divulge anything.

Tuesday

Arrange for a box of chocolates to be sent to your lovee that day. Attach a note on the beautiful stationery that coordinates with the previous invitation. Address the note to her middle name and write, "Enjoy these chocolates or save a few to share during our weekend together. Don't share them with anyone else—keep this gift a secret, as we mustn't get caught. Be careful: don't let anyone know of my invitation or our weekend away. Your husband [enter your first name] mustn't know. I can't wait to be with you. More details later. Love . . ." and sign it with your middle name. The element of secrecy heightens anticipation and a sense of excitement. She'll be incredibly, deliciously curious about what you have planned, but willing to indulge you and keep the secret because of her burning curiosity.

Wednesday

Send her a pair of matching scented candles with another note on the stationery. Address it to her middle name again, and write, "Bring these with you on Friday when we meet, so we can make love by their light. Meet me Friday at 6 p.m. at [describe your meeting point]. Tell your husband [insert your first name] that you need to go away this weekend on unexpected business. Love ..." and sign your middle name. If you've chosen a hotel in the city where you live, tell her to meet you in the lobby of the hotel. If your destination is further out, tell her to meet you at the train station (give an exact location), or give her a place to meet you where you'll drive up in your car and pick her up. Later that night, when she tells you that she's going away for the weekend (and can you please take care of the children), simply agree amiably and innocently, and give her a kiss on the cheek.

Thursday

Have a gorgeous, sexy shoulder bag delivered to her with your note inside. Once again, address it to her middle name and write, "Pack everything you need for the weekend in this. Don't let your husband [insert your first name] see it. He must suspect nothing. The weekend is ours to share. I'm counting the hours before I can see you, touch you, kiss you. Don't forget: tomorrow, 6 p.m. sharp. Love ... " and sign your middle name. That night, give her some time alone so she can pack without interruption or discovery.

Friday

In the morning, send her a beautifully wrapped box containing lingerie. Attach a note that says, "Be wearing this under your outfit when you see me this evening. Remember: 6 p.m. tonight. [State the meeting place]." At some point in the day, confirm with the concierge your arrival time and make sure that, before you check in, your room is decorated with flowers, and stocked with wine and cheese. Ensure that the wine and cheese are waiting for you in your room, as a post-check-in room service delivery will run the risk of you being interrupted in flagrante delicto. For an extra-special touch, make sure that the wine and cheese match. You may ask the concierge for their recommendations, or consider pairings of:

Brie	Cabernet sauvignon
Camembert	Pinot noir
Gruyère	Pinot noir
Feta	Chardonnay
Chèvre	Sauvignon blanc

Meet at 6 p.m. and check in to the hotel; when you arrive in the room, don't pause for breath before pushing her up against a wall and kissing her. Hang the "Do Not Disturb" sign on the door and make love immediately. Let the wine sit and sweat in the cooler while you act like a lover who has hungered for her for weeks. After you've rumpled the sheets, open the wine and enjoy it together, luxuriating in the hotel bathrobes. When the doorbell rings, ask her to answer it and then watch her face as she realizes it's another invitation. This invitation, handwritten by you, should read, "The pleasure of your company is requested at [insert your chosen restaurant]. Tonight. Love ... " and sign your middle name. Smile at her when she looks up, and say, "Meet in the lobby at 8 p.m.?" Change and leave her to dress. While she's dressing, go out and confirm that the restaurant has received the bouquet of red roses you arranged with the concierge. Make sure they will have them wrapped in a ribbon and on the table when you arrive.

Enjoy your evening out together, and when you arrive back at the hotel, make love again. Choose sexual positions that you don't regularly engage in, to differentiate this weekend from your usual sex life and emphasize the idea that you are two slightly different people making love, in a fresh seduction.

Saturday

When the (prearranged) room service breakfast arrives, with a flower and another invitation, make sure she opens the envelope while you're in the shower. The invitation should read, "Meet me at noon at [choose place]. Love [your middle name]." Enjoy the morning together and suggest that maybe she'd like to do some shopping before your rendezvous. Meet her at noon for a lunch, or a stroll through a park or a museum, or any number of activities that you don't normally do together. By continually using invitations, despite being together for the whole weekend, you cement the theme, and it is one of playfulness and surprise, confirming the weekend as an affair between your alter egos. It also shows an attention to detail few long-term couples display when romancing each other. Most couples might surprise their lovee with a weekend away, but not continue the surprises throughout the entire two days, or play along with the theme the entire time.

As the afternoon wears on, ask your lovee if she'd like to go back to the hotel room for an afternoon delight. Make love all afternoon, enjoying each other nude without any other obligations, except to be together. Tell her how much you appreciate this stolen time away together. Order room service for dinner and don't feel the need to go anywhere at all. This weekend is about time shared together, with no pressure to sightsee or charge around discovering a new place, because it's secret, treasured time alone, just the two of you.

Sunday

Enjoy your last morning together in any way that pleases you both, and before you check out present her with a parting gift: a picture postcard of the hotel, framed. Tell her to open the frame and see that you've secretly written her a love note on the back, addressed to her middle name and saying something like, "With memories of our secret, stolen moments together on [enter dates of the weekend]. With love ... " and sign your middle name. Tell her that when she gets home she's to put the frame somewhere special in her house, and to think of the love note secretly hidden on the back, in the frame, whenever she looks at it.

Go your separate ways at the original meeting point, and give her a passionate farewell kiss, as if it were a kiss to end all kisses.

Extra Zing

On Sunday, add another gift to the framed hotel postcard. Give her a second postcard of an exotic destination, and on the back write that you've planned a romantic week away for an overseas holiday for the two of you. According to research, the top ten most exotic, erotic and romantic destinations in the world include:

1. Amalfi Coast, Italy
2. British Virgin Islands, Caribbean
3. New York, USA
4. St Petersburg, Russia
5. Seychelles Islands off the coast of Madagascar
6. Prague, Czech Republic
7. Rajasthan, India
8. Fiji, South Pacific
9. Barcelona, Spain
10. Iceland

Do your own research to choose your personal most-romantic destination if any of these top ten destinations aren't appealing to you.

Tell her to keep this postcard in her lingerie drawer, as an enticing initial invitation, and to look forward to future invitations and love notes detailing this next getaway together . . .

Gourmet

Come sit naked,
relax,
make this almost perfect
when every whisper would beg,
tease.
We did always like
that language.

A Toast and a Tipple

New Year's Eve

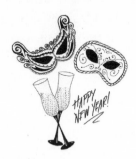

Pleasure Pantry Ingredients
Formal wear
New Year's Eve party hats
Frozen lemonade
Pineapple juice
Sparkling lemonade
Gin
Grenadine
Lemon or lime slices
Champagne
Champagne flutes—2
Dinner or party reservations (optional)
Fondue set (optional)
Cheese (optional)
Chocolate (optional)
Romance-themed stationery (optional)
Erotic book (optional)

Preparation
New Year's Eve: a time to celebrate. Take this evening to celebrate not only the coming year but each other, and your relationship and love. Amidst all the hustle and bustle of the

festive season, make sure you take some time to prepare for your loving and passionate New Year's Eve by getting all the necessary ingredients and making the plans and reservations (if required) well in advance, including preparing your toasts to each other. Decide together whether you'd like to spend the night out or in, then plan as appropriate. Come New Year's Eve, indulge in each other and toast to your love and a new year together.

Bring to Boil

Regardless of whether you're staying in or going out for the eve, dress up for the occasion—even though you know you'll be dressing down, and off, soon enough. Celebrate the tradition and formality of the event of New Year's Eve by dressing sensually and sexily in formal wear, to embody the romanticism of the evening. Dress up attractively for each other, from the inner wear out, to get in the sexy mood of enticing each other into a whole new year as a loved-up couple. Top off your outfits with New Year's hats—after all, when else do you get to pair formal wear with cardboard and sparkly tinsel? Maximize the theme of the evening by going all out, even if you're staying in.

Save the champagne for later, and instead start the eve with a kicker cocktail. Create a taste for the New Year with the lip-smacking zing of a citrus cocktail of New Year's Eve Punch made from a classic 1965 recipe. Blend slightly frozen lemonade, pineapple juice, gin and a splash of grenadine together, and garnish with a slice of lemon or lime.

If you're going out to a New Year's Eve party, make sure you find a few moments together, quietly just the two of you, for a private toast to each other before midnight. If you opt to stay at home, arrange for a hot, sexy evening in focusing on each other rather than the TV telecasts of NYE celebrations. Wink to the past with a New Year's dinner of retro-chic fondue. With a fondue set, you can enjoy cheese and/or chocolate fondue, seductively feeding each other and licking dribbled bits off each other's chins and fingers. Deliciously sexy!

About thirty minutes before midnight, grab a bottle of champagne and pour each other a glass; take turns toasting each other. The key to this year's NYE toast is to freshly differentiate it from any other toast you've ever given to your lovee, and celebrate them for who they are now, as you look towards a future year together. Bear in mind that most people make strict and stringent New Year's resolutions every year, about how they must be better, do better, eat less, exercise more, cut out vices ... et cetera! So use your toasts this year to neutralize the negative New Year talk.

Toast your lovee with how beautiful and wonderful they look, and are, and describe everything you love about them, everything they do well, everything they've accomplished that year, your memorable highlights of the year, and your favorite memories shared with them that year. Make them feel loved inside and out, and celebrate how fabulously fantastic they are, just as they are here and now, tonight. After you've both toasted each other, clink glasses and cheer to another year together. Then, at the stroke of midnight, passionately kiss. Give your lovee a deep, loving kiss that invites them into a promise of another amazing year to share with each other.

Anytime after midnight, whether it is 2:30 a.m. or 7:30 a.m., make love to initiate yourselves into the new sexy year.

Make love as a couple who can't get enough of each other, a couple who desires each other at every waking moment. There is a common belief in many countries that dictates that how you welcome the New Year signals how that year will be for you, so make it hot and loving. Start your New Year off with a bang. Create private and passionate fireworks that will stay with you all year long.

Extra Zing

To add extra spice and sparkle to your year ahead, make a passion pact of New Year's sex resolutions. Every January the 1st, most people make New Year's resolutions for every aspect of their lives—except their bedroom life. This year, each of you make a pact for six sexy New Year's resolutions. But not resolutions, really—make them New Year's sex desires for the coming year. Each of you come up with six things you'd like to personally experience in the next twelve months— romantic, spicy and detailed fantasies to have fulfilled, ways of making love, or dream locations to do it in . . . The only rule is that they have to be doable in the year. For example, don't write, "Take me to Brazil for sex on the beach" if an overseas trip is beyond your budget for the year. Make your resolved desires practical, but passionate and pleasurable.

Take the New Year as an opportunity to write down the things that you'd most love to romantically and sexually experience with your lovee that you haven't ever experienced or shared yet, or at least in a long while. Whatever your wish list, both of you individually write each of your six sexual desires on six separate pieces of lovely, romantic, erotic stationery that you've chosen and purchased together, and read them to each other on New Year's Eve as a primer to tease each other for what will be coming in the New Year. Randomly shuffle them, and slip each piece of paper between different pages of the erotic book that you've bought. Put the book in your bedside table drawer. Once a month, take the book out and read the erotic stories to each other. When you get to a page containing a piece of paper describing one of your desires, start to plan how to enact that desire as soon as possible that month. Then continue reading the interactive book each month, until twelve months have passed, all twelve of your desires have been fulfilled and another New Year, and new future, has arrived.

Flirtini for Two

Valentine's Day

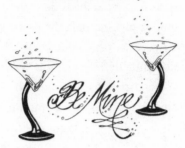

Pleasure Pantry Ingredients

Flirtini cocktails:
   Stolichnaya Razberi vodka
   Cointreau
   Lime juice
   Pineapple juice
   Cranberry juice
   Raspberries
   Brut champagne
   Sprigs of mint
Love notes or cards
Chocolate
Gift coupon for lingerie
Gift coupon for a CD
Flowers
Hired limousine and driver
Loose flower petals (real or silk and fabric)
Picnic hamper of finger food & sushi
Flirtini glasses—2 (optional)
A variety of flirtatious, loving gift coupons—11 (optional)

Preparation

Valentine's Day, February 14, is one of those dates in the calendar of a couple's life when sex is most definitely on the menu. But many couples expect it so much that some of the creative, gourmet pizzazz—roses, chocolates, card, champagne, dinner, sex—gets left out of the seduction of the day.

This year, give your Valentine's Day a slight spin on seduction. Don't take each other's romance and love for granted: flirt a little. Inject your love life with the same kind of invigorating flirtatiousness as you had when you first started dating and expressing your new-found love for each other.

Most people think of flirting as something one does with a stranger, or else only at the blossoming beginning of a relationship, to be quickly replaced by the surety of love and established connection with each other. But the fun and games can continue in a relationship. Flirting releases endorphins in your bodies, immersing you in surges of titillating responses which make you feel good. Just because you're in a steady relationship, that doesn't mean you can't still flirt with each other and remind yourself why you fell head over heels for your lovee, and how you're still falling for them every day.

Plan a scavenger hunt in order to seduce your lovee playfully on Valentine's Day. Send them on teasing, pleasing errands led by flirty, encouraging notes. You may both like to play this game with each other, or one of you may like to surprise the other. Instead of champagne and roses this year, twist it with Flirtinis and a limousine littered with petals of all different types and colors.

To prepare, ensure you make all the arrangements well ahead of time. Because Valentine's Day is excessively busy for almost all businesses in the romance trade, you need to pay extra attention to detail by discussing your plans with each shop manager and the limousine company weeks ahead. Make sure you get the flower petals ordered well before the day, and the ingredients for the Flirtinis. A Flirtini has Stolichnaya Razberi vodka, Cointreau, lime juice, pineapple juice, cranberry juice and a few raspberries muddled in the bottom of the glass, topped with Brut champagne. It can be garnished with a sprig of mint.

The Flirtini is a drink that was conceived for Carrie on *Sex and the City*. It's not only sexual innuendo in a glass, a fun touch for the night, but is sweet, smooth and seductive in taste. The Flirtini also has its very own glass, designed to complement the drink, and you might like to order a pair from a boutique glassware company or an online shop, to drink from in the limo and really encompass the excitement and unique celebration for the night. Ask the limo company to have the Flirtini ingredients and glasses ready in the car for when you are picked up (or, if you're surprising your lovee this night, you can arrange this yourself). They can be packed in a picnic basket or red-themed cooler, along with the flower petals scattered around the limo seats and floor. If the limousine company objects to fresh flower petals because they may ruin the upholstery or leather interior, choose a selection of silk or fabric petals instead. They won't let off the same aroma, but they can still have the same effect.

Prepare for a night of flirtation and seduction, not only as a romantic couple in love, but a couple who flirt with each other and show each other how lustful and fun being together can be ...

Bring to Boil

Flirt (verb): to make playfully sexual or romantic overtures.

Start your February the 14th by defining the day with a flirty morning kiss (a hint that loving things are in store for your lovee today) and a wink and a smile. During the day, send your lovee flowers and/or a card or love note containing the first playful errand for them to run on. In the note, direct them to the chocolate shop you have chosen to pick up something sweet. Tell them it's there waiting for them; all they have to do is go into the shop and ask for the message in their name. When they go to the chocolate shop, they'll be given a large handmade chocolate with your message iced on top of it. It might be "I love you [name]" or "Be mine," or any traditional or non-traditional sentiment you've chosen to have the chocolate decorated with.

Wrapped in with the chocolate is a second love note, and another flirty mission. In the note (accompanied by a gift certificate), direct them to a second place: for her, it may be a lingerie shop; for him, it may be a music store. Tell her to pick out lingerie of her choice to wear tonight; tell him to pick out a CD to listen to—and make sweet love to—tonight. He can be given the choice, or a list of top ten sexy or romantic CDs may be included in the note.

When they pick up this second special present, cashing in the gift certificate, the salesperson at the store should then hand over another love note in an envelope (it's important to have this prearranged with the store by coding the gift certificate with an oblique reminder for the salesperson to do this). This third love note directs them to a particular florist, where they then go to pick up flowers already ordered and waiting for them. Attached to the flowers is a handwritten note from you, stating where and when to meet that night. Choose as the destination one of your favorite places, such as your favorite beach café, bar or restaurant.

When they arrive to meet you with lingerie on (underneath clothes, of course) or CD in hand, take their hand and give them a kiss. Lead them out onto the street, where a limousine is waiting. Invite them into the limousine, where flower petals cover every inch of the inside and you have Flirtinis waiting. Ask the driver to put the new CD on and instruct them to simply drive around town so you can take in the lights and sights.

You may like to go to various special and romantic spots that mean something special to the two of you—you could drive past the restaurant where you had your first dinner date, the place where you first kissed, places filled with memories of romantic encounters of the past, places where you celebrated previous Valentine's Days ... Circle the city, luxuriating in the limousine—a vehicle of romance itself—playing with seductive body language, paying each other compliments, talking, laughing and simply enjoying each other's company.

Open the picnic hamper and feed each other dinner of finger food or sushi. You might like to stop the limo and set up the picnic in a park, or eat inside, never leaving your private love cocoon—until you're dropped off at home, where sex in your bedroom is guaranteed now that you've flirted your way into each other's hearts all day and all night.

When you make love, tease each other: touch each other through your clothes; take a long time to make out before getting undressed. Flirt with each other in bed, kissing and whispering, "Do you want more?" "Shall I touch you here?

What about there?" and "Can I have you now? Will you be mine?" Cupid doesn't need arrows tonight. A little fun and thoughtful attention is all it takes.

Extra Zing

One of the reasons some people don't like Valentine's Day is that it can feel contrived: just one day when romance is obviously on the agenda, and when the pressure of making romantic gestures and giving demonstrative gifts seems overwhelming. Some partners and couples would rather ignore Valentine's Day than deal with that external pressure for public expressions of private feelings. Or they staunchly believe that they show their lovee how they feel all the time, on other nonspecific days which aren't scripted.

However you feel about Valentine's Day, it's important to show your loved one passion, romance, flirtation and affection—and not only on one day per year. To spice up your romantic life beyond February the 14th, secretly arrange for eleven gift coupons, whether they are personally handmade; sexual, romantic or indulgent in nature; for travel, sporting or little fun trinkets. They should be delivered to your lovee on the 14th (or another day if you object to the 14th) of each month for the rest of the year. Show them that they are your Valentine every month, and that you treasure them all the time, not just on one marked day of the year.

Be mine? Oh, yes please. Today, tomorrow and always.

Breakfast at Tiffany's

Her birthday

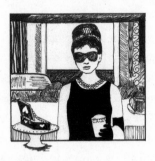

Pleasure Pantry Ingredients
Single flower
Present from Tiffany's wrapped in their classic turquoise blue box
Birthday card
Cash or credit card (yours)
Formal wear
Dinner reservations
Tickets to the ballet, symphony or theatre
Constellation certificate
Custom-made pendant (optional)

Preparation
Give her a star-studded bling-bang birthday treat this year. Start her day with a thoughtful breakfast that you cook or order yourself, making sure to include her favorite breakfast foods—fruit, muffins, etc—and Tiffany's present. Then shower her with attention and gifts all day, indulging and spoiling the woman who is the star in your life.

To prepare for her birthday surprises, make sure you've chosen something from Tiffany's and bought her a card, flowers, and tickets to a show that you know she'll love and feel spoiled by; that you've made dinner reservations and arranged to have a star in the sky named after her. Research one of the companies which do this (there are a few easily found on the internet), and then enjoy the sparks as they fly . . .

Bring to Boil

At midnight, as the clock ticks over to her birthday, wake your lovee by tickling her shoulders and chin with the petals of one flower. When she wakes, kiss her gently, give her the flower, wish her a happy birthday—wanting to be the first to do so—and tell her that you're taking her out to breakfast first thing in the morning, to celebrate her birthday. With a smile and a kiss on her shoulder, give her a loving light back rub, soothing her back to sleep, and let her drift back into dream time.

In the morning, wake her up with tea or coffee placed on her bedside table, with one flower in a vase next to the cup. Kiss her happy birthday (again) and invite her to get showered and dressed, ready to go out for a birthday breakfast. Take her out for coffee and croissants (if you're both working that day, squeeze in the time for an early breakfast together before work). Present her with a Tiffany's box during your breakfast together. Even with a tight budget, just about anyone can save to buy a gift from Tiffany's. You can get her a stunning piece of jewellery or a simple yet beautiful bracelet or keyring. Whether it is small or substantial, a woman always feels classically and romantically spoiled receiving anything from Tiffany's encased in their traditional turquoise blue box and bow.

At the end of breakfast, give her a birthday card in which you've written that her birthday surprises continue, because you're taking her out for a day of shopping. If her birthday falls on a work day and both of you can't get the day off work, arrange for the shopping day to occur the next Saturday. Otherwise, grab her hand and lead her to a day of splurging.

Take her first to one of her favorite clothing shops and ask her to find a dress that she'd like to wear tonight, for a glamorous night out. Get her to try on many dresses and outfits, à la Julia Roberts in Pretty Woman. Sit and admire each fitting and twirl until she chooses what she likes best. From there, take her to a shoe shop for the same indulgent treatment. Continue taking her to a variety of shops, but once she's chosen a dress and pair of shoes, at each shop thereafter you should alternate who gets to choose what for her. At the next shop, perhaps a perfume shop, pick out a fragrance for her. Then at the next place, perhaps a beauty shop, she can pick out something. Not all shops have to be expensive—the indulgence of the day is in spending it shopping together, lavishing attention on her. Take her to a florist, a Dollar Shop, drugstore, beauty store, housewares shop, a chocolate shop, an accessories shop ... Make it a game in which you both have fun, but the attention is squarely focused on her as the birthday princess.

Once you have totally indulged her with a dream shopping spree, take her for coffee at a plush café or afternoon tea at a lovely traditional hotel where they serve high tea. Here, tell her that her birthday surprises aren't over, but that the day's shopping has really been a primer for the elegant evening you have planned. Let her know that she has the rest of the afternoon to get dressed and made up for a stylish and chic night out, just the two of you. Tell her what time she needs to be ready, and leave the rest as a surprise.

When you're both formally dressed, including you in a tuxedo (rent one if you don't own one), let her in on the secret that you're taking her out for dinner and a show (whatever you've chosen—ballet, symphony, theatre—musical, etc).

Enjoy your romantic, elegant dinner for two, and at the end, have the waiter bring her a special birthday dessert, with one small but tasteful birthday candle to blow out, before going to the show.

Afterwards, don't head home straightaway but, rather, draw out every minute of your classy evening together, making the most of the night to celebrate her and why you love her so. Invite her for a walk, taking her to a secluded spot where you can gaze up at the stars without distraction or disruption. Point out constellations and beautiful stars in the sky. Tell her that she's more beautiful than all the stars in the sky. Then face her, and say to her that you want to show your everlasting admiration and celebration of her, so you've had a star named for her. Kiss her, then raise her eyes to the sky and point out exactly where "her" star is. Take out the con-stellation certificate as confirmation that you've named a star for her, and give it to her, promising to frame it for her. Tell her you've chosen that particular star for her because it's always visible on her birthday, and because it reflects how you feel about her: singular, unique, bright and everlasting. Kiss her under the stars, and with the star-bright love you feel for her.

Take her home, kissing her at every possible second, showing her your love, feelings and desires effusively. Lead her into the bedroom and lie her down against the bed; but rather than get undressed immediately, stay partially clothed in your elegant wear. Hike up her gown, slip off her panties and go down on her. Let her experience your hot tongue on her as she's still wearing her formal dress, and make her feel like she's so irresistible to you that you can't even wait to take off her dress before kissing and pleasuring her. Please her to a peak under her satin, silk and tulle before coming up for air, to fully undress her. Make love to her, whispering and calling out her name, over and over, focusing all your attention on her. Afterwards, wrap the both of you in the bed sheet and lead her over to the bedroom window to gaze back out at the stars. Point again to the one that is named for her. Tell her that, even though her birthday is nearly over this year, her star shines bright, like your love, for ever immortalized.

Extra Zing

For an added special touch on her birthday, have a piece of jewellery made just for her. Have a gold or white gold (whatever her preference is) square pendant made, engraved as a calendar month, detailing the month of the year she was born. In the date of her birth, have a small diamond set. Tell her it's a unique commemoration of her and her birthday, and it's hers to wear every birthday from here onwards. Whenever she wears it, on birthdays to come or on other days, she'll always think of you and your thoughtful celebration of not only when she was born, but who she is and what she means to you.

A Feast for His Eyes Only

Birthday. His birthday.

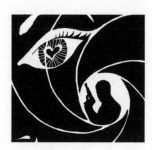

Pleasure Pantry Ingredients
Classic bacon and eggs breakfast for two
Birthday card (James Bond theme)
Adrenaline-pumping extreme experience gift certificate. Choose one
    from a selection, such as:
        Jet adventure flight
        Vintage flying
        Helicopter flight/lessons
        Acrobatic flying
        Flight simulator
        Skydiving
        Parasailing
        Scuba diving
        Porsche power experience
        Rally car experience
        High-performance supercar driving experience
Tuxedo or other formal wear
Retro 1960s-themed lingerie
The birthday boy's favorite dinner
Dry vodka martinis
Martini glasses—2
Birthday cake
Music soundtrack of a Bond film (his favorite if he has one)
Handy-cam video camera (optional)

James Bond-themed party decorations, food, drinks and costumes
  (optional)
James Bond DVDs (optional)

Preparation
Bond together on his birthday by giving him an elite,
extreme experience of the James Bond ilk. To prepare,
arrange the adventure of his dreams as a surprise. Plan the
day so that it's an exciting adventure culminating in a swish
dinner of his favorite fare and a sultry night in.

Give him a pumping great birthday to remember—a
thrilling ride, complete with his very own Pussy Galore.

Bring to Boil
Start off the birthday boy's morning by getting onto his
Morning Glory. If you have children, lock the bedroom door;
strip him down to his birthday suit and make love to him in his
favorite position. When you've both worked up an appetite,
cook a breakfast of scrambled eggs and bacon—simple, but a
favorite of James Bond's, and it sets the theme for the day. Kiss
him happy birthday and give him his birthday card over breakfast. If you can, find a James Bond-themed card or, if not, find
one with a picture hinting at the day's adventure, but don't
present him with the gift certificate yet—give him a chance to
be surprised later in the day. Tell him to dress in appropriate
attire, without revealing too much about what you've planned.

Drive to the venue and enjoy the look of excitement on
his face as he realizes what he's being treated with today. It
might be getting to race around a track in a high-performance
supercar, learning to fly a fighter jet, skydiving, flying in a
vintage plane or acrobatic flying lessons—any high-performance, high-adrenaline, boy's-toy, grandly dangerous

and awesome Bond-type adventure. Ideally, you can share the adventure together. Couples who take risks together, who simultaneously feel the rush of adrenaline by stepping outside their comfort zone, can reinvigorate their passionate relationship by recapturing that amazing thrill, the kind of zing and excitement you felt when you first started to fall in love with each other, when nothing was sure and everything about being together felt like heady, crazy sparks shooting straight down into your heart. Many of the extreme-adventure options can be bought as a gift certificate for two. However, if you're not a risk-taking kind of person, invite his best mate to come along and enjoy it with him instead. You can then watch and cheer your man on, and take a handy-cam home movie of him experiencing his high-speed, high-thrill adventure. Give your filming James Bond-type commentary, perhaps even using famous movie lines, or boosting your man by comparing him to the legendary James Bond. Admire his form. He's your legend.

In full adrenaline rush, at the end of the day's adventure, take him home for more 002 time. As he's showering, place an outfit for him to wear on the bed (a tux is the obvious option, of course, but any formal wear will do), and you can take this opportunity to change into a new, yet unseen by him, set of lingerie with a 1960s feel to it. It might be a sheer babydoll negligee, or an outfit similar to that worn by one of the many Bond girls in any of the films. In your lingerie, and nothing else, cook his favorite dinner. Give him a feast for his eyes as you prepare the meal; this is very Bondesque. Be a woman who exhibits herself seductively, near nakedly and obviously unabashed in the presence of such a suave and dashing man. Flaunt your sexuality for him in a powerful, seductive way.

As the meal is cooking, start your evening with—what else—the Bond drink of choice: a medium-dry vodka martini. Shaken, not stirred.

As you sip your martinis, and then enjoy your dinner, flirt wildly with him, liberally using sexual puns and innuendos (the cornier the better) to enhance the mood and have fun with the "Bond"-ing. For dessert, present him with a birthday cake decorated in either the Bond or extreme-adventure theme. Enjoy feeding each other pieces and, when you're ready to escalate to a sweeter seduction, take some of the leftover cake with you to the bedroom. Top off the night as James Bond would, naturally, with a saucy sex session. James Bond always makes time for plenty of sex between his missions and adventures, so sex twice in one day is not only following the Bond example, but is also a birthday treat times two.

Slinkily drop the top half of your lingerie and dip your finger into the frosting of the leftover birthday cake you've brought into the bedroom, coating your nipples with it. Drop them into his face to lick clean. Play with the birthday cake, eating it off each other, spreading it over both of your bodies and nibbling it off. After you've finished with the serve of birthday cake in the bedroom, pull your leading man onto you and kiss him while uttering a classic Bond girl quote: "I think I will very much enjoy serving under you."

Serve your birthday boy well, until The End.

Extra Zing

Host a swanky James Bond 1960s spy-themed surprise birthday party for him, in his honor. Invite all your and his friends and family with 007 Birthday Mission invitations, and ask them to dress in 1960s sexy formal "James Bond" or "Bond girl" costumes. Do your Bond research and cater for the night using all the clichéd but classic Bond ingredients. Supply martinis, Bond food featured in the various films (fan websites are dedicated to meticulously recording these to ease your menu planning), play Bond film soundtracks as background music, and decorate the house with Bond movie posters. Even have a supply of Bond DVDs playing on mute on the TV screen as an added thematic touch.

Classic Bond drinks recipes should include:

Medium-dry vodka martini
(from *Dr No*)
2 oz vodka
$^1/_2$ oz measure of dry Vermouth
Shake well with ice and pour into a martini glass. Add a thin slice of lemon peel.

The Vesper
(from *Casino Royale*)
3 measures of Gordon's gin
1 measure of vodka (preferably a Russian grain vodka)
Half a measure of Lillet Blanc
Shake very well until ice-cold. Pour in a deep Champagne goblet and add a large, thin slice of lemon peel.

Americano
(From *Casino Royale* and *A View to a Kill*)
1 oz Campari
1 oz Cinzano Rosso
Perrier

Put the ice in an old-fashioned glass. Add the Campari and Cinzano, then pour in a splash of soda water. Add a large slice of lemon peel.

Black Velvet
(from *Diamonds Are Forever*)
1 part Guinness Stout
1 part chilled champagne
Add the Guinness to a pint glass and pour the champagne on top.

At your suitably chic cocktail birthday party, among family
and friends, give your dashing man a public Bond birthday
toast, from his number one Bond girl, and raise a glass ...
(and, as Bond might say, raise something else—a little more
privately—later!).

Milk Maiden

Mother's Day

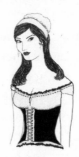

Pleasure Pantry Ingredients

Chrysanthemums—white
Mother's Day present or gift hamper from you and the children
Mother's Day card
Tulips—red and yellow
Irises—yellow
Roses—mauve
Sexy, loving, non-Mother's Day card
Massage vouchers for 2
Gift certificate to a deluxe day spa
Picture frame (optional)

Preparation

Mommies are more than milk-laden mammaries. Moms, with their wonderfully voluptuous boobs and bottoms, are hot, sexy mamas too. It's important to make your partner feel like a desired, irresistible woman and your adored lovee, not only mother to your children, on Mother's Day and every day. As the mother of your children she is, of course, vitally important and intimately connected to you. However, many partners, especially over time, get into a routine of being co-parents to their children and focusing on domestic issues, building a solid family foundation together, so that treating each other as passionate lovers can fall into the background or be relegated to harried moments of "when we can find the time and we're not too tired."

On this Mother's Day, shower the woman in your life with your ardor. Appreciate her not only as a mother but your partner in life and love, too.

To prepare, you need to buy flowers, presents (with the children), book masseurs and, most importantly, arrange with family members to look after the children for a few hours in the afternoon, after you have a family Mother's Day lunch or celebration. Whatever you have to agree to do in return, do it, because you want some treasured alone time hours on this day to cherish her as a mother and especially as a lover. Your lover. Make your milk maiden feel like a MILF (Mom I'd Like to Fuck).

Bring to Boil
Engage in the traditional morning ritual of bringing Mum breakfast in bed, and present her with a bouquet of white chrysanthemums, the traditional Mother's Day flower. Enjoy the morning in bed, sharing it together as a family. Give her your Mother's Day present and card—the ones that can be shared in the company of the children.

Even though the Mother's Day present has to be tame, that doesn't mean it has to be tedious. Do not give her a toaster. Do not give her a blender. Do not give her slippers. Frankly, she can buy those items herself. Domestic goods and comfy footwear don't speak as loudly in the lusciously appreciative stakes as, well, just about anything else. Get creative; make sure your present is sweet and has a tiny, sexy teasing tinge to it.

Don't be afraid of a little bit of affectionate play in front of the children. They know it's a special day to honor Mom, and many children feel reassured by seeing some affection between their parents (sometimes also step-parents, depending on the situation). Regardless, children like to see their mother loved and appreciated by all of you, and that goes especially for her loving partner too. It's good for them to see this bond between you.

Build a tailored gift hamper for her around a theme or color. Work with the children to come up with the idea and scour the stores with them for little and bigger gifts that fit your chosen theme. Involving the kids in this way is fun, and they'll be itching to give her the present and see her open it that morning.

After the initial morning ritual, shoo the kids out of the bedroom (send them to clean up the kitchen after preparing breakfast!) by telling them it's time for Mom to shower and change. When the kids are gone, tell her that you have some special, secret and private celebrations for her today, and the first one is waiting for her in the bathroom. Let her go in to discover a second bunch of flowers waiting for her, with a sexy card attached. The flowers you choose can be any which have a personal romantic connotation, or that you know are her favorites; or you may like to arrange red and yellow tulips, with yellow irises and/or lavender roses. For the message you want to convey today, above and beyond loving her as a mother to your children, these flowers are particularly appropriate. You might like to work their meanings into the message you leave on the sexy card for her.

Each flower represents something and for these it's: our love is pure (lavender rose); my love for you is passionate (yellow iris); you are a perfect lover (red tulip), and, I am hopelessly in love (yellow tulip).

After your Mother's Day obligations and celebrations with each of your mothers and/or extended family, leave the children with relatives as prearranged. It's perfectly acceptable on Mother's Day to steal a few hours alone as a couple, especially once you've had the traditional gift-giving and quality family time.

Lead your love maiden back to the house with a cheeky grin. She's going to expect that you've taken her back to slip in a few hours of sex. You have—but not yet. There's still a surprise in store.

Tell her she's about to be pampered all over her body, expertly. When the masseurs arrive, enjoy a lovely relaxing massage, side by side. (If you can't arrange for two masseurs to come to your home, you can alternatively check yourselves into a day spa that caters to couple massages, if not that day then on another day you have planned and booked.) Once you've both been spoilt by relaxing aromatherapy massages, whisper to her to stay naked as you show the masseurs out the door and welcome in some treasured alone time.

Come back to her and kiss her from her shoulders across her breasts, up her neck and full on her lips. Make love to her in the kitchen, on the table, on the floor, and seated up against the kitchen benches. Have needy, loud, uninhibited sex, sure in the knowledge that the kids cannot interrupt you, shifting from place to place in the house. Lead her into the laundry and have sex against the washing machine, or with her sitting up on its edge (maybe even as it's on spin cycle!). Eroticize every part of your house that seems associated with domestic work. Sear memories into her brain of being naked together, sexing up where you usually do the dishes and sort the whites from the colors.

Afterwards, bask in the glow of the afternoon light and your lovemaking. Enjoy this cherished time together, alone as a couple, before returning to your children and the world of parenthood.

Extra Zing

To make her feel extra special, give her a gift certificate to a day spa. Make sure she knows that you'll take care of all the details, including childcare, so she can have the entire day free for pleasure and pampering. Send her off to a day spa that specializes in all the luxuries like mud wraps, milk baths (excellent for skin softening) and floral-scented facials. Tell her to indulge in re-energizing her whole beautiful body.

You might also give her a really special memento that celebrates her both as a mother and a lover. Buy a gorgeous picture frame with as many windows in it as you have children. Go through your photo albums and place in the frame copies of photos from each day that she gave birth and held her babies for the first time. Arrange them together in the frame according to the order of births, and have the frame engraved with a personal sentiment, for example, "As the mother of our beautiful children, I love you. As the partner in my life, I love you even more." *Mamma mia!* She'll be very touched.

Sugar Daddy

Father's Day

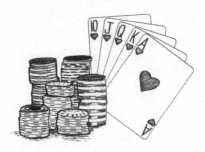

Pleasure Pantry Ingredients
Father's Day present from you and the children
Father's Day card
Men's ties—2 (new)
Romantic, loving, non-Father's Day card
Deck of cards
Poker chips
Sexy, saucy, non-Father's Day card
Lingerie (new)
Beer
Cigars
Powdered sugar

Preparation
He's the daddy—give him some sugar. Have some fun celebrating your man as the father of your children, but raise the
stakes to indulge him as your manly stud by teasing him
with a little strip poker on the night of Father's Day. Doing
this isn't just playfully adding spice to your sex life together,
but also shows him very blatantly, and very nudely, in a
saucily rude way, how sexy you think he is, how much you

desire him and just what it is he does so well ... that made him a dad in the first place!

Prepare by getting all your ingredients ready well ahead of time, which includes not only buying the presents and poker-themed gear but also brushing up on how to play Five Card Draw and Five Card Stud.

Bring to Boil

Enjoy your Father's Day together, with all your family traditions, including presenting him with a gift you and the children have selected or made, and a heartfelt card about why this is a special day to show your love and appreciation for him as a great dad. In the morning, make sure you steal a moment to get him alone to give him your private, personal presents, to celebrate him as the main player in your life. Give him a box with two nice ties in it—ones you know he'll love wearing. Attach a romantic card in which you express how much you love him, and adore and appreciate him as the father of your children. When he's thoroughly grateful, and gives you a thank-you kiss, pull back from his lips with a smile and tell him, "But wait, that's not all!" Then give him the flirty present to hint at what's to come that night. Wrapped in red and black wrapping paper, give him a deck of cards (naughty nude ones) and a stack of poker chips. On the sexy card write something deliciously teasing and playful like, "Ready to gamble with your clothes? Place your bets tonight. 9 p.m. Bedroom. You, me, Strip Poker. Winner takes ALL! I'll give you a head start—wear the two ties I gave you."

At 9 p.m., after the kids have gone to bed and you've had a fantastic Father's Day together meet in the bedroom. Now it's "down and dirty, delight Daddy time." Wearing your new sexy lingerie that he hasn't yet seen under your clothes, pour two mugs of beer and light a couple of cigars, to embrace the poker night theme. Sexily wrap your lips around the cigar and suck, looking at him directly with a flirty wink.

Agree to the rules you're going to play by and sit on the bed across from each other. Deal the cards and begin playing each hand. Someone must strip at least one item of clothing at the end of each hand. Get into the play by betting big and bluffing wildly. The goal isn't really to win—it's to lose … your clothes and his.

When you're both nearly naked and flushed, take the two ties you bought him (that he's lost and discarded in the previous hands), and use them for the real purpose you bought them for: to tie him up and say, "I win. And you win."

Tie him up gently (because men's ties aren't ideal for knotting around wrists, tie them loosely so they don't constrict or hurt him). Straddle him and kiss him. Make him feel like he is absolutely not in control—you're the dealer, and the feeler. Rub your body up and down his. When he is ragingly hard, get on top and ride him as you also stimulate your clitoris with one of your hands. Show him your hand; tell him to watch you touch yourself as you fuck him. Slow down your rhythm as you begin to approach orgasm, so that, just as you're about to explode with pleasure pulses, you can pump up and down on him hard and fast to get both of you to come at the same time. Fold down onto him, completely spent. Untie him and drape the two ties on his chest. He'll remember this playful night every time he wears either of them. Just what you were betting on! Ace.

How to play Strip Poker

While Five or Seven Card Stud may sound sexier, when it comes to Strip Poker for two, Five Card Draw is the simplest—and most effective—game to play. Basically, both players ante up, meaning they each place a small bet in the middle pot as a starting betting point. Ante-up chips in strip poker can be kisses, as the base for each round, so that not only does whoever wins see the other strip an item of clothing, but they win the same amount of kisses as chips were thrown in for the initial ante.

The dealer then deals each player five cards, alternating cards and starting with the other player. Each player looks at their hand to check out what they have. The other player bets first, followed by the dealer. Players can (but don't have to) trade in one, two, three or four cards to try to improve their hand and strengthen their bet. With new hands, each player bets more.

In Strip Poker, bets can be represented by poker chips, but you say out loud what item of clothing you're betting. One might say "I bet my top" as they toss in a chip. The other might respond with, "I'll bet my pants ... and raise your bra," meaning that they're raising the stakes so that if you accept and play on (otherwise folding and forfeiting your top), should you lose you must strip your top and also your bra. Continue the betting until someone calls "Reveal," and then each player must show their cards. Best hand wins. Loser loses their clothes, and winner takes in the seductive view and accepts the winning kisses.

Winning hands

Royal Straight Flush: 10, J, Q, K, A all of the same suit.
Straight Flush: five cards of the same suit, in order.

Four of a kind: four of the same card in each suit (5, 5, 5, 5).

Full House: a set of three of a kind, plus a pair.

Flush: five cards all of the same suit, but not in any order.

Straight: five cards in a row, by number, but not of the same suit.

Three of a Kind: three cards of the same number or rank.

Two pair: two pairs of the same number or rank, such as a pair of fives and a pair of sevens.

One pair: two matching cards, such as two Kings.

High Card: if neither of you has any of the above winning hands, the player with the highest card in their hand wins. Ace high. Ace in the hole!

Extra Zing

Up the ante of your strip poker game by betting not just clothes but powdered sugar 'body shots' as well. Each time one of you loses a hand, not only do you remove one article of clothing (or allow your playmate to remove it for you), but anywhere your playmate's skin is showing, pour a sprinkling 'shot' of powdered sugar on it and then suck it off. At first, this might be on their lips or neck, but as you each get more and more revealing, lick and suck breasts, navel, ankles, backs of their knees and upper thighs ... until you're both nearly completely nude and your sugared-up loving leads you to each other's sweetest spots.

Mmmm. Everyone wins.

Merry Merry Cherry

Christmas

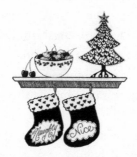

Pleasure Pantry Ingredients
Red stockings decorated with cherries and love hearts—2
"Naughty and nice" sexy Christmas boxers and lingerie
Cherries
Brandy
Brandy snifters
Cherry chocolates
Hot chocolate
Cherry-tart-flavored lube
Sexy love coupons
Cherry-themed notepad or stationery
Santa hat
Cherry-themed panties and bra (optional)
White cotton G-string and bra (optional)
Cherry iron-on transfers (optional)
Red cherry or love-heart love notes (optional)

Preparation
Christmas is a holiday which can bring not only much joy, but also a fair amount of stress too. Couples try to fit the end-of-year work in with seemingly endless shopping for relatives and friends, a large pile of Christmas cards to

get into the mail on time, the exhaustive party circuit and food and boozy celebrations, and sometimes strained deliberations about "where to spend Christmas Day this year." Amidst the hectic scheduling and harried shopping, it's important to take time out for each other during the holidays. While Christmas is an annual family holiday, acknowledge yourselves not only as people who are part of a larger family but as a close twosome too. Celebrate the year spent together, and your private connection as a couple, as the year winds up.

Whether you're having a cold, white, snowy Christmas or a hot, red, sunburned holiday, steal a few quiet moments away from the holiday cacophony and chaos to kiss and cuddle, and to play "naughty and nice."

To prepare for these stolen moments together on Christmas Eve, try to be as organized as possible come December 24, with all the shopping done and at least most of the presents and stocking-stuffers bought and wrapped. If you're still up at 2 a.m. building a dollhouse or putting a tricycle together, you'll be too tired and too busy to play hotly and sweetly with just each other. So it's worth spending a few late nights earlier in the month wrapping gifts and assembling tricky children's items from Santa. That way, after the kids have gone to bed on Christmas Eve, you can play your own saucy version of Santa and Mrs Claus.

Bring to Boil

'Twas the night before Christmas and all through the house, not a creature was stirring ... so go have sex!

Take advantage of those few precious hours of deep sleep your children experience (if you have them), before they come bouncing onto your bed before the crack of dawn, wanting to open the presents under the tree. To avoid the risk of being discovered by children, you might consider playing in the bedroom; otherwise, make love by the tree, celebrating the sexier spirit of Christmas and giving each other memories to last all through the morning present-opening ritual with family and friends there. Blushing memories. Hot memories.

Take the private, sexy Christmas stockings you decorated earlier for each other, giving each other the only rule of using a red and cherry theme, and then open them together, first admiring the creative, sexy effort that was put into the outside of the stocking before plunging in. The presents you give each other should be fun, naughty and red-hot-and-juicy-cherry themed. If you wish, you can agree earlier in the month, as you plan this night, to limit your spending budget to a set amount, laying down the challenge to each other to get creative and sexy with only one limitation to your sexual imagination.

Start by giving each other "naughty and nice"–themed boxer shorts and lingerie—and insist on putting them on right then, to continue your gift-giving and receiving in the near nude. It is, after all, the perfect night to wear a pair of briefs that say naughty on one side and nice on the other. Which is it? Or maybe it's a little of both this year?

Presents you might give each other could then start with a bag of cherries. Eat some this night as you continue to play. You might also like to sip on some randy brandy in large, voluptuous brandy snifters, as you exchange gifts, to loosen the mood and complement the cherries. While brandy can be regarded as a sexual disinhibitor, cherries are considered an aphrodisiac because they contain vitamins A and B, which aid in the production of sex hormones, and also zinc, which is good for sperm production. Love is a bowl of cherries!

Other presents might include cherry chocolates (another aphrodisiac); a package of hot chocolate with a note attached promising to enjoy it in bed together later, as a sexy postcoital cuppa; a cherry-themed bra and panty set, which can be expensively bought, or else buy a simple white cotton G-string and T-shirt bra, and iron transfers of cherries bought from a craft shop. At the tip of her stocking, right down at the bottom, he can add a tube of cherry-tart-flavored lube, and write a note to her saying, "For my sweet tart. For you to put on ... and me to take off." She can give him a book of sex coupons, or she can even make them herself on red sheets of paper decorated with cherry and love-heart stickers. Each of them could be for one wish fulfilled whenever he chooses, such as "This certificate entitles you to one nude weekend," or "Present this coupon to redeem one red-hot blow job, anywhere you choose, anytime you want," or "For a good time, call [the fantasy character of your choice] and I'll be her for you." One of you could also give your lovee a red or cherry-themed notepad, and on the first page quote one of the most famous love poets, Pablo Neruda: "I want to do with you what spring does with the cherry trees." Oh my!

Flushed and ripe for sex, strip down and make love in the nude, except for him wearing his Santa hat. Lie on top of him and playfully tease him as "Saint Dick." Take a few cherries and tantalizingly suck on them, making your lover watch every lick of your tongue and squeezing smack of your lips as you wrap them around the soft, wet skin of the deep red cherry. Feed them to each other and smear cherry juice down each other's chins and chests. Fuck either in the fiery, searing heat of the summer or in front of a fireplace in the freezing cold of the winter, and fuck with a crimson, luscious desire.

Extra Zing

Leave your lovee hot and juicy love notes on red paper, cut out into hearts or decorated with cherry stickers, all around the house for them to find on each of the 12 days before Christmas. Use these as reminders to lead up to your hot and oh-so-private Christmas Eve celebration. Tell them sweet thoughts in the notes, or give them hints about what you're going to do to them that special eve.

If you don't celebrate Christmas, no matter what your culture or religious belief, this can still be a fun way to tease each other at the end of the year, and to focus secret attentions on each other during the holiday season.

Joy to the world. Joy to you and me!

Salsa Love

Your anniversary

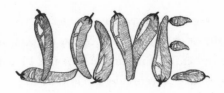

Pleasure Pantry Ingredients
Voice-recording alarm clock
Anniversary presents
Anniversary cards
Flowers (red and yellow)
Latin Love Recipe creamy long cocktails—2:
   Coconut rum
   Banana rum
   Pineapple juice
   Raspberry
   Coco Lopez cream of coconut
   Cream
   Ice
   Coconut shavings
Blender
Gambas al pil pil (prawns, olive oil, garlic and chillies)
Oversized cocktail goblet
Dagoba xocolatl organic chocolate
Chilli-themed cocktail napkins
Chillies
Chocolate dipping sauce
Photo album
Dinner reservations
Salsa lessons

Hurricane glasses—2
Photographer or artist (optional)
Photographs of you two on your honeymoon (optional)
Brightly colored pieces of paper and brightly colored markers
   (optional)
South American–themed room decorations (optional)

Preparation

Give your anniversary a hip-swivelling south-of-the-border feel this year. Prepare all your goodies and memories, and sizzle together as you celebrate another year notched up, and more to come. Celebrate how you met and fell in love, and the details of the history of your relationship, before heating things up with a salsa lesson, and then a rumba between the sheets.

Bring to Boil

Start the morning of your anniversary by waking up to a voice-recording alarm clock (available at novelty shops and online boutiques) on which you or your lover has prerecorded an anniversary message, introducing a touch of the theme, and welcoming them into the day of your anniversary by saying something such as "Hola my hot tamale. Happy anniversary. I remember when we first [choose a first thing you'd like to recall as you're waking up together in bed, such as a first kiss, first time you made love, first danced as a married couple at your wedding]. And I remember when I first laid eyes on you. *Fue amor a primera vista* [It was love at first sight]. Wake up, wake up, *mi amante, alma mia di corazon. Te amo* [my lover, dearest of my heart. I love you]."

Later you can re-record over and over on the voice-recording alarm clock, so that during the times over the coming year when one of you may be on a trip, you can leave love messages for your partner to wake up to; or else have them on special days, and other times when you just want to give them a sweet start to their day.

To start your anniversary day, exchange gifts and cards over breakfast. Depending on the year of your anniversary, you can choose a gift according to the traditional wedding guide:

First	Paper
Second	Cotton
Third	Leather
Fourth	Books
Fifth	Wood or clocks
Sixth	Iron
Seventh	Copper, bronze or brass
Eighth	Electrical appliances
Ninth	Pottery
Tenth	Tin or aluminum
Eleventh	Steel
Twelfth	Silk or linen
Thirteenth	Lace
Fourteenth	Ivory
Fifteenth	Crystal
Twentieth	China
Twenty-fifth	Silver
Thirtieth	Pearl
Thirty-fifth	Coral or jade
Fortieth	Ruby
Forty-fifth	Sapphire

Fiftieth	Gold
Fifty-fifth	Emerald
Sixtieth	Diamond

During the day, have a bouquet of red and yellow flowers sent to her with a floral card featuring a sexy note, or a chilli image as decoration. Emphasize the South American theme by choosing flowers that are very bright, as red, yellow and green are the colors of South America, and most of its nations' flags.

Spend all day sending your partner sizzling emails and text messages so they become primed for the night. When you are finally home, change into sexy salsa dancing outfits. Before heading out for a celebratory evening of Latin lovin', share a few moments in, quietly just the two of you. Blend together a few creamy cocktails of Latin Love Recipe, a long, sexy drink renowned for its seductive connotations. While one of you blends the drinks, the other can put together an *aperetivos* (appetiser) of *Gambas al pil pil*, a traditional South American starter of king prawns cooked in olive oil, garlic and fresh chillies. Place the prawns (Latino prawn cocktail style), hanging over the edge of a very large cocktail goblet, the inside of which is filled with fresh red chillies as decoration and outside has been kissed with red lipstick lip imprints. Add sex and spice to your starter: "Spice a dish with love and it pleases any palate" (Plautus, c254–184 BC). Scatter broken up pieces of Dagoba xocolatl chocolate around the base of the oversized cocktail glass and on the chilli-themed cocktail napkins. "Dagoba xocolatl" is a South American chocolate made with cocoa, chillies, vanilla, nutmeg and maca, and is available to order online. Also add chocolate-covered chillies (seeds scooped out prior to dipping in chocolate). These can be for thematic decoration, or the brave can try a crunch!

As you sip on your lover-ly drinks, and enjoy a taste of the sexy South, surprise your lovee with a gift of a photo collage in an album or frame, celebrating all your "firsts," big and small. Or else you can surprise them with the gift of a photographer or artist to come and take your portrait, perhaps in a special locale, such as where you married or where you had your first date; or arrange to have a picture taken of you dressed up and salsa dancing, to commemorate how you spent this anniversary night.

Go out for dinner at a South American restaurant. If there isn't one conveniently located near you, a Spanish tapas restaurant can also give a similar flavor and ambience. Then dance the night away after taking an introductory salsa lesson at a club. If you've never danced the salsa before, try it together tonight, as a first, creating another new 'first' memory as a couple.

Sweaty and exhilarated, and very turned on to each other after all that sexy dancing, go home and make hot—sizzling hot!—love to each other. A fucking fiesta! Olé!

Extra Zing

Decorate your bedroom as a surprise for your lovee, around the theme of your honeymoon to remind you of when you first married; but to make it a little different, give it a spicy tinge. Add some heat to the remembrance of your honeymoon, rather than a straightforward reminiscence and reflection.

If you honeymooned in a beach destination—even if it

wasn't a South American island or coastline—create an ambience for the night around a hot and sexy beach theme, complete with a colorful Mexican hammock strung up above your bed as a canopy. Or if you honeymooned in a cold, snowy locale, add to your wintry theme with Peruvian wool blankets and the vibrant colors of South America. Convert your bedroom into a visual ode to your anniversary, your wedding and where you honeymooned, with a fiery enthusiasm and zest for details.

In addition to your Latin lovin' theme, place copies of photos of you and your lovee on your honeymoon all over the walls. Intersperse them with brightly colored pieces of paper on the wall, which feature loving dedications and declarations to your lovee, as well as cherished memories you have over the year(s) of your relationship. Write things like, "Remember when we first made love?" or "Remember the time when we …" and post memories of all the places you've been, things you've shared, as well as everyday times you've laughed and loved. Twist the theme further with a South American beat by having salsa music playing in the room, and dance in each other's arms, holding each other close, at the foot of your bed. Embrace your salsa love. And your spicy sex.